Sleep Better to Thrive

Practical Steps That Will Enhance Your Life

Dr Sui H. Wong MD FRCP

Table of Contents

Introduction

Sleep affects everything.

What comes to mind when you think of health? Perhaps you focus on food, or maybe the image of an athletic person pops into your head. However, one foundational aspect of your health that should not be ignored is your sleep habits.

Almost every living animal sleeps. Some get a lot of rest, like koalas, which can sleep for 18 or more hours a day ("Koala," 2020). Others, like giraffes, sleep less than five hours a day (Suni, 2023a)!

Sleep can be an overlooked area for those looking to self-improve and feel better. The more serious effects of poor sleep aren't felt as immediately, and the less serious effects can be masked with things like caffeinated drinks or sugary snacks. Chances are, you've heard someone say, "I can sleep when I'm dead," or maybe you've said it yourself!

In reality, sleep deprivation will likely shorten your life *and* affect your productivity. How many times have you stayed up late even though you knew you had to wake up in the morning? When was the last time you hit snooze and slept in for more than 20 minutes past your intended wake time?

Like other aspects of our health, many of us know that we might need to improve in this area, but the problem is knowing how to go about getting more high-quality sleep. Throughout this guide, you will follow a step-by-step process to improve your sleep quality for better overall health.

To kickstart your journey toward better sleep, we'll start by discussing the importance of setting a consistent wake-up time every morning. This simple habit will help you establish a healthy routine, understand your sleep needs, and avoid building up a sleep debt. You'll discover why it's crucial to wake up at the same time every day, even on weekends, to regulate your body's internal clock and improve your sleep quality.

After that, you'll fine-tune your nightly routine by determining the ideal bedtime based on your target sleep duration. For instance, if your goal is seven hours of sleep, you'll learn how to adjust your routine accordingly in a seamless and practical way to align with your body's natural rhythm. By the end of this journey, you'll get to know your sleep needs and optimal sleep patterns, and you'll learn strategies to enhance your sleep quality.

Quality sleep isn't just crucial for brain health resilience; it's essential for productivity, health, and overall well-being. This workbook aims to empower you with practical tools for establishing and maintaining healthy sleep habits!

A Note From the Author

As a neurologist (medical doctor) and neuroscience researcher in interventions to improve brain health, I understand the importance of sleep for your health. I have experience in clinical applications to treat medical and neurological conditions and have used my skills to support successful behavior change.

I frequently assist those interested in improving their sleep patterns. Changing sleep can change lives in many ways, such as by reducing migraines and boosting daily alertness. In addition, many people transition from feeling foggy to feeling clear and refreshed daily. With these practices, it *is* possible to see amazing results that will change your life for the better.

My motivation to write this book comes from the questions and challenges I often see in my clinical practice. The approaches throughout this book include many things that have been helpful and effective in improving the quality of life of my patients. Now, I'm looking to share this expertise with a wider audience so more people can have a positive impact on their lives beyond my day-to-day clinics!

I'm passionate about the importance of sleep, and I have witnessed firsthand the negative impact that a lack of sleep can have on health. It's my mission to transform people's health in my medical practice.

I aim to convey kindness, compassion, empathy, and motivation in my approach. My goal is for individuals to feel empowered and inspired to take positive steps. While the journey may seem challenging at times, persisting and following the process will bring valuable rewards!

As we begin, I want to encourage you to reflect on your underlying motivation—your profound "why." This might include the desire to improve, to support your family, to be a better partner, sibling, or teacher, or to excel in your professional roles.

Take a moment to write your "why" below. What are your goals, and what motivates you to improve? Writing this down will help you reinforce this idea:

_____

_____

_____

_____

Then, throughout the process of sleep improvement, you can return to this motivation to help you stay focused and on track with your goals. Identifying sources of joy, purpose, and significance is key to making a positive and long-lasting change!

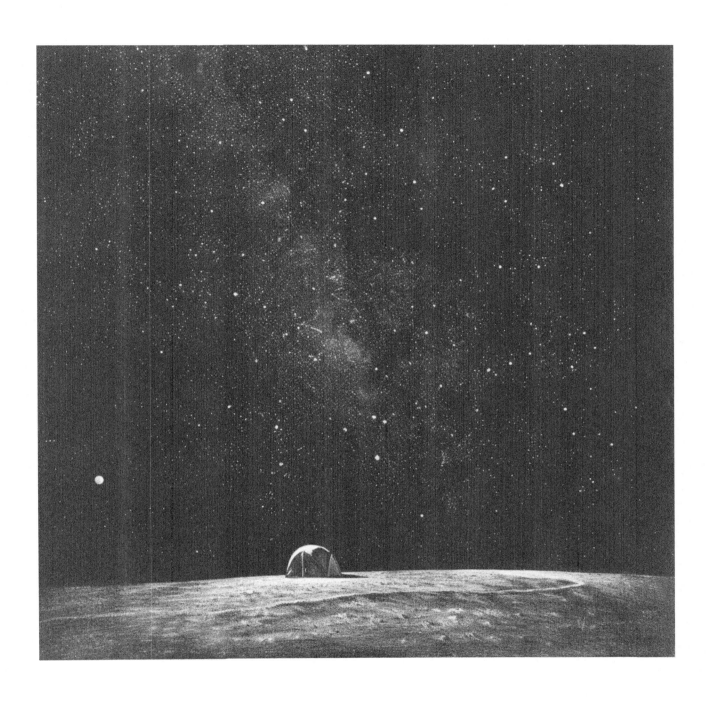

Chapter 1:

Health First—The Science Behind Sleep

Knowing the science of what is involved when your body goes to sleep will help you understand why it's important to create a routine, and how you can troubleshoot sleep issues.

Throughout the next six chapters of this book, you are going to learn everything you need to know about sleep quality and how to perfect your routine. By the end, you can take what you've learned and apply it to your life so that within a few weeks, you will notice an improvement in the quality of your sleep. At the end of the book, in the additional resources section, you will find an action plan that you can then implement to help you take the right approach to your health.

You already know sleep is important, which has inspired you to come here! Now, let's take a deeper dive into why it's so vital for your health and what's going on inside the body during this restful period each night.

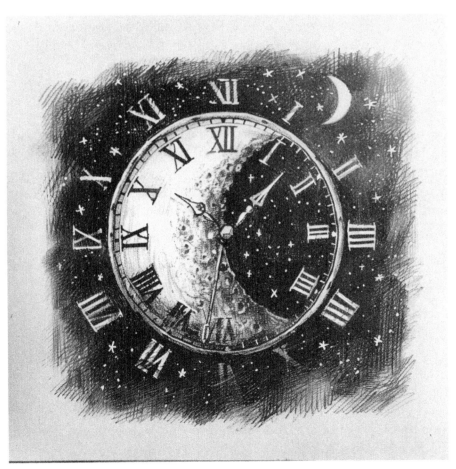

The Importance of Sleep

Sleeping is something we've been doing since we were born—and even before that! When in the womb, it's estimated that fetuses are sleeping about 95 percent of the time (McTigue, 2020). Sleep isn't a practice you have to learn how to do; our bodies are naturally wired to send signals of tiredness and alertness throughout the day. However, what we *do* have to learn is how to maintain consistent and regular sleep. Why is that? Below are some FAQs to help you understand what sleep is, why it's necessary for your body, and why sleep regularity is important for overall health.

Why Do We Need Sleep?

Sleep, in its simplest form, is a restorative process. Consider any part of your body, whether it's your heart or your stomach. Every area needs some form of rest. Nothing ever stops working completely, or else it wouldn't function properly. However, not everything works at a rapid pace all day long. You can only run so far until you need to stop and catch your breath to give your lungs a break. You can only eat so much until you need to stop and let your stomach digest. You can only stand so long until your leg muscles need rest and you have to sit down.

The brain needs rest, too, just like any other part of your body. It never stops working, but sleep is an essential process that helps your brain increase neurological functions, such as (Bryan, 2023):

- learning

- memory

- immunity

When you sleep, your brain is working hard to help improve and regulate everything going on in your body, from digestion to hormonal balance.

What Does a Lack of Sleep Do to the Body?

According to the National Heart, Lung, and Blood Institute, "The way you feel while you are awake depends in part on what happens while you are sleeping" ("Why Is Sleep Important," 2022).

Poor sleep health is associated with (Carden et al., 2021):

- cancer

- cardiovascular disease

- diabetes

- increased mortality risk

- obesity

It's clear to see that poor sleep health contributes to these things, and it exacerbates any other health conditions you may already be struggling with. Failing to provide your body with proper sleep may be just as detrimental to your health as poor nutrition, lack of physical exercise, or excessive stress.

What are Some Misconceptions About Sleep?

One of the biggest misconceptions about sleep is that your body can adjust to poor sleep. At times, it might feel like it. Perhaps you only slept for three hours before a big day at work, and you ended up feeling fine after some coffee and a cold shower. These things only mask the symptoms—they don't remedy the problem. This can make it feel as though missing sleep isn't a big deal, but doing so on a consistent basis could lead to poor health later on.

Another misconception is that how much you sleep is the main thing to consider and that napping will supplement your sleep. It's true that napping can help you feel restored, but it is not a replacement for healthy sleep (Suni, 2023c). In addition, it's not true that the more sleep you get, the better off you will be. While getting an adequate amount of sleep is important, what's more important is that the type of sleep you're getting is high quality to ensure your body is experiencing that natural restorative process needed.

What are the Stages of Sleep?

Chances are, you've heard of the stages of sleep. At the very least, you've experienced what they feel like! Each night, our bodies go through different stages of sleep, each serving a different purpose ("Sleep," 2023). Each stage takes your body into a deeper slumber as it progresses, and your body cycles through all of the stages four or five times a night. The cycle usually lasts between 90 to 120 minutes. The four stages of this cycle are:

- NREM (non-rapid eye movement) stage 1

- NREM stage 2

- NREM stage 3

- REM (rapid eye movement) sleep

The non-rapid eye movement (NREM) stages begin when your body starts to fall asleep.

During the three stages of non-rapid eye movement, your body starts the process of falling asleep. In stage 1, you might easily wake up as this is a light stage. During stage 2, your brain is more relaxed and your brain waves slow. Then, in stage 3, you enter deeper sleep, your brain waves slowing even more as the restorative process kicks in.

Lastly, during the REM stage, your brain actually becomes more active, and this is the stage when you're most likely to dream. During each cycle, the REM stage becomes longer.

Why is it important to know about these stages? In order to get a full night's rest, your body needs to cycle through these stages multiple times to help organize information, store memories, and restore your body's energy. If there are disturbances that cut a large percentage of stage 3 sleep at night, such as caffeine or alcohol use, you may be deprived of the benefits of that phase, such as flushing toxins.

In addition, this helps explain why naps can sometimes be counterproductive. If you sleep long enough to enter NREM stage 3 and then wake up, you might feel groggy and confused ("Sleep," 2023).

Since each REM stage becomes longer throughout the night, if you have to wake particularly early one day for something like a flight, then it's the majority of the REM phase that will be affected. In this case, making small schedule adjustments leading up to the trip may help you get more sleep to prepare.

Understanding these sleep stages teaches us that sleep is a complex process, not just a quick resting period for your body. Improving sleep requires that we learn how to work with the body to facilitate deeper, restorative sleep to improve the way we feel during the day.

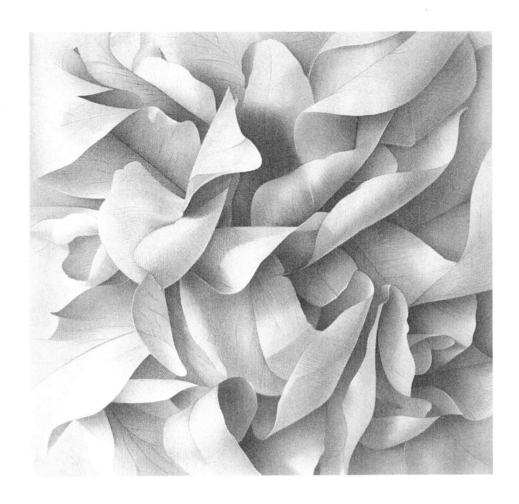

How Does Poor Sleep Affect Productivity and Concentration?

Another key thing to know about sleep is that it is a chemical process in the body. Each stage produces hormones that are vital to help the body function (Suni, 2023b). When you sleep, your brain goes through cognitive processes, such as (Suni, 2023b):

- memory consolidation

- clearing out dangerous proteins

- connecting and strengthening ideas

When we skip these cognitive functions, it will make it harder for our brains to work properly during the day. Memory recall becomes more difficult, impairing our ability to think logically, problem-solve, and follow directions. When our ideas are disorganized, it may be less productive and struggle to carry out important tasks.

Aside from the biological processes that we miss out on during poor sleep, grogginess can lead to impulsivity, and fatigue will reduce motivation, therefore impacting our daily routines.

Why Does Disturbed or Unregulated Sleep Cause Emotional Dysregulation?

As previously mentioned, missing out on sleep impacts various cognitive functions, which will also influence how you manage emotions. Sleep deprivation can make us more sensitive to stressors and reduce our ability to cope with emotions (Vandekerckhove, 2017). When you are not getting enough sleep to support cognitive baselines for your health, you will end up struggling with additional life pressures.

Think of it this way: If you live a sedentary lifestyle, doing basic forms of physical activity might be challenging, such as walking up several flights of stairs or standing for long periods of time. On top of that, additional physical activity, like participating in a sport, is going to be even harder.

When your brain isn't getting enough sleep, you won't be providing it with the baseline of rest needed for the natural restorative process. Then, any additional life demands that bring on stressors of their own become even more challenging to deal with. Excessive stress also takes your body through a chemical process, dysregulating your hormones.

A lack of sleep can cause stress, and stress can cause a lack of sleep, thus contributing to a cycle that leaves you feeling tired, burnt out, and overwhelmed.

How Does Sleep Deprivation Impact Metabolic Health?

It's clear to see how and why sleep deprivation impacts the mind since so much happens during sleep, cognitively speaking. But now you might be wondering how this impacts your body as a whole.

Since so many hormones are released as you fall asleep, during sleep, and upon waking, that means your body relies on hormonal balance for proper function. Once your sleep hormones are disrupted, the impact will spread to other hormones that regulate blood sugar, hunger, and blood pressure. This could lead to cravings and overeating habits, disrupting digestive health even further.

On top of this, your overall metabolism is disrupted when poor sleep habits take over, impairing the body's ability to regulate body weight. All of this reduces energy, which could lead you to crave high-calorie foods or sugary, caffeinated drinks as your body seeks sources of energy. In turn, this impacts your weight even more, thus contributing to a cycle of unhealthy sleep.

Troubleshooting Health Issues

Sleep is the keystone habit that promotes other healthy habits, like getting the right nutrition and physical activity. While it might not appear that way at first, there are many symptoms you may be struggling with that are related to your sleep habits.

Take a moment to reflect on some of the things you've been struggling with in terms of your health. Below is a chart that encapsulates some of the biggest health issues related to poor sleep quality. Make a note of any you are experiencing, along with the symptoms you've been dealing with. You might find that you just haven't realized sleep contributes to them!

Common Health Issues	Symptoms You May Be Experiencing
Emotional Dysregulation	<ul><li>mood swings</li><li>anxiety</li><li>depression</li></ul>
Lack of Motivation or Low Productivity	<ul><li>procrastination</li><li>poor work or school performance</li><li>struggles with task completion</li></ul>
Trouble Focusing or Concentrating	<ul><li>struggles with paying attention</li><li>memory issues or forgetfulness</li><li>trouble listening or comprehending information</li></ul>
Weight Management	<ul><li>slow metabolism</li><li>obesity</li><li>sudden and unexplained weight loss or weight gain</li></ul>
Metabolic Health	<ul><li>intense food cravings</li><li>high blood pressure</li><li>irritability</li></ul>
Lack of Energy	<ul><li>lethargy</li><li>fatigue</li><li>bursts of energy followed by energy crashes</li></ul>

Sleep Assessment

Once you've established the more important reasons for taking care of your sleep health, you start to create better motivation to stay on top of these habits. It can be difficult to make habits and lifestyle changes if you don't first understand why it's necessary to do so. Getting better sleep is good for obvious reasons, like feeling more refreshed and reducing grogginess. However, it's what's going on inside of the body that is key in regulating your total health.

Next up is a self-assessment to help you lay the groundwork for your own personal sleep routine. Take some time to reflect on the questions below. Use the lines provided to write out your responses, or write them in a separate lined notebook if you're using an eBook.

What makes it hard for you to regulate your sleep patterns?

_____

_____

_____

What are the biggest things keeping you from sleep?

_____

_____

_____

What habits do you knowingly participate in that might be making it difficult to sleep?

_____

_____

_____

What are your biggest strengths when it comes to keeping a sleep routine?

_____

_____

_____

What in your environment is keeping you awake?

_____

_____

_____

How are your stress levels?

_____

_____

_____

What are your other healthy habits like, such as eating habits or workout routines and exercise regimens?

_____

_____

_____

Now, using the answers you provided above, fill out the chart below, or copy this template into a lined notebook if you're using an eBook. In the left column, some examples have been provided for you. Use a pen to cross off the ones that might not be an issue for you, and use a highlighter to mark the ones that you do need to work on. In the right column, write your own responses. Use bullet points to help you focus on the most important things keeping you from healthy sleep.

The things preventing me from maintaining a regular sleep routine are:	<ul><li>anxiety</li><li>nightmares</li><li>waking up in the middle of the night</li><li>poor habits, such as phone use before bed</li></ul>	My response:
The biggest disruptions I have when sleeping include:	<ul><li>noises, such as a partner snoring</li><li>getting up to urinate frequently</li><li>uncomfortable sleeping situations</li></ul>	My response:
The habits that are hardest for me to break when it comes to regulating my sleep health are:	<ul><li>staying up later than I should</li><li>sleeping in later than I should</li><li>drinking caffeine close to bedtime</li></ul>	My response:
When it comes to getting regular sleep, I'm best at:	<ul><li>going to bed at the same time every night</li><li>getting the same amount of sleep every night</li><li>following a solid nighttime routine</li></ul>	My response:

There are some factors outside of my control that disrupt my sleep, such as:	<ul><li>outside noises, such as traffic or noisy neighbors</li><li>light disturbances due to irregular shift work</li><li>pets or kids who disrupt my sleep</li></ul>	My response:
When talking about my stress level and the biggest stressors that keep me from getting better sleep, I would probably say:	<ul><li>financial issues</li><li>work-related stress</li><li>family or relationship issues</li></ul>	My response:
I would describe my eating habits by saying:	<ul><li>I eat fairly healthy and am satisfied with my dietary choices</li><li>I eat mostly healthy, but could use some work</li><li>I don't eat very healthily and could use some improvement in this area</li></ul>	My response:
I would describe my physical activity habits by saying:	<ul><li>I exercise frequently and consistently</li><li>I exercise occasionally but could use some more physical movement in my routine</li><li>I rarely exercise or get much physical activity at all</li></ul>	My response:

Chapter 2:

Routine and Rhythm—Crafting Your Sleep

Routine

Have you ever wondered why we sleep during the night and are awake during the day? Do you know why some animals come out at night and others are only active in daylight? Nocturnal animals who sleep during the day and are awake at night have natural functions built into their biology that assist with survival at night. Humans, on the other hand, are diurnal, and rely on sunlight for optimal performance.

Because of artificial light and the hectic demands of daily life, humans are less reliant on the natural cycle of the day, which can contribute to problems with sleep. Within us all, we have a circadian rhythm that tells our body when to conduct vital bodily functions, such as releasing hormones and hunger signals.

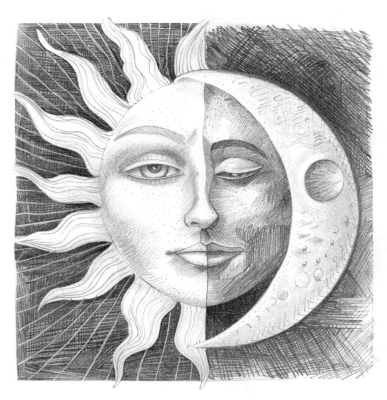

Understanding Circadian Rhythm

For most species that aren't domesticated, this circadian rhythm depends on the sun and moon. Both provide light signals, or lack thereof, that indicate when an animal should wake up and start the day. Humans, on the other hand, often depend on alarm clocks and other disturbances to rouse us from sleep. But that doesn't mean we don't still have this biological wiring within us.

What Is a Circadian Rhythm?

The circadian rhythm is a 24-hour cycle (Bryan, 2024b). Throughout the day, as the sun changes, so will your sleepiness. When it's bright in the morning, this alerts your brain to feel awake. As the sun sets and night comes, this tells your brain it's time to wind down and head to bed. This is helpful on a biological level for many reasons. It helps conserve energy and regulate bodily functions, like digestion. Our metabolism fluctuates throughout the day to ensure we aren't constantly hungry, and at night, your metabolism slows to preserve energy while you're sleeping.

This is just one example of the many processes that occur in your body each night. Your brain has a main biological master clock, the suprachiasmatic nucleus (Bryan, 2024b). Why is it important to know about this? The more regularly your rhythm aligns each day, the easier it will be to regulate your body, thus supporting normal energy and metabolic functions. We encounter many disturbances throughout the day, like stress or eating, that can impact our circadian rhythm and contribute to feelings of sleepiness.

How Does Light Impact Sleep?

Since the sun is such a vital signifier for many bodily functions, light can disturb your sleep. Ever wondered why your eyelid skin is so thin? This is so that even when we close our eyes at night in the dark, we can still sense light signals. We've all been in a room, fast asleep, when someone comes in and turns on the light. Though our eyes are closed, this still signals to the brain that light has appeared, thus inducing wakefulness.

When sleeping, it's important to have a dark environment that helps remind the brain that it's time to rest. We can't always follow the exact cycle of the sun—you might work late at night, requiring you to sleep later in the morning than when the sun rises. Even when we don't naturally align with the changes in the day, we can still create environments that support a healthy circadian rhythm by creating the proper light environments. Tips for the right lighting will be discussed later in the book, but for now, it's important to touch on just how much light impacts our ability to sleep.

What Hormones Are Involved in Sleep?

Throughout the day, various systems within us work hard to regulate our bodies through hormones. Sleep plays a major role in hormone regulation. Humans have more than 50 hormones responsible for maintaining our health ("Hormones," n.d.). Let's take a look at a few specific ones:

- **Melatonin**: Melatonin is one of the most important hormones for sleep, and actually controls over 500 of your body's genes (Vinall, 2021)! This is first released when darkness is sensed, which is why we get sleepier at night. It's also released during sleep, enabling you to stay asleep.

- **Human growth hormone**: Growth hormones are released throughout the day but peak during sleep. This is essential for regulating your metabolism and is especially important in children's growth ("Human Growth Hormone," n.d.). One study showed that those with post-traumatic stress disorder (PTSD) experienced sleep disturbances that impacted their growth hormone levels (Hong, 2015). This shows the impact that the mind has on the body, and how stress, sleep, and metabolism are all interconnected.

- **Cortisol**: Though known as the stress hormone, cortisol is involved in energy regulation. Cortisol can provide your body with a feeling of alertness, which is why it's related to stress. When your body perceives a threat, this signals cortisol release, helping you become more aware of your surroundings and ready to take action. However, it's also released daily to help manage your alertness. Cortisol release goes down at night, then peaks in the morning (Stanborough, 2020).

As you can see, sleep disturbances can cause issues for your energy, hunger, and stress levels. When hormones are disrupted at night, that will have an impact during the day, and vice versa. For example, if you're overly stressed throughout the day, this might cause an excessive release of cortisol, which could make it hard for you to fall asleep.

What Is Sleep Pressure and Adenosine?

Adenosine is a chemical that regulates your sleep drive (Bryan, 2023). This determines how energy is stored or used in the body, and also helps with basic functions like muscle contraction. During the day, adenosine builds up, just as our desire to go to sleep does. Once we reach a certain level of adenosine in our brains, we're given a signal that it's time to go to bed. Then, as we sleep, adenosine is reduced, just as our sleepiness is. Adenosine and the circadian rhythm work together to support your sleep cycle.

This helps us understand sleep pressure and our ability to regulate energy throughout the day, and it explains why we feel more tired as the day progresses. However, when those signals telling us to go to sleep are ignored, it can impact our brain's functioning. This is why you might find it hard to focus and concentrate when working or studying late at night. Though you might be fighting sleep, your body is working hard to signal to you that it's time for rest.

Why Is It Important to Follow a Routine?

Due to the light fluctuations on Earth, the hormones in our bodies, and the natural passage of time, our bodies depend on a routine to help us function. When we have dysregulated schedules, this disrupts the body's ability to function.

Think about the last time you learned something new. Maybe this was a new job, or perhaps a hobby. The first few times you tried this, you likely had to put more energy into focusing and doing everything right. You triple-checked your work and read instructions twice to ensure you did it all correctly. The more you did this, the easier it became to complete tasks.

In a sense, the body relies on this same kind of regulation. When it can prepare for everything during the day and follow the same patterns, it's easier to maintain hormonal balance and helps your bodily systems conduct business as usual. When your schedule is dysregulated or you aren't getting adequate sleep or nutrition, your body has to spend extra energy making up for these deficiencies, while also trying to maintain regularity.

When this occurs, it starts to throw off your entire hormonal system, therefore triggering additional stress or poor eating habits. You might find that it's hard to focus on work or you have intense food cravings. If you miss work or overeat, you might feel stressed about this, further disrupting your hormones. It might make you feel tired, so you try to sleep more, but this only disturbs your sleep and leads to more stress.

Having a few nights of poor sleep here and there isn't the end of the world—the body is resilient and can adjust. However, when irregularity is the norm, it creates a cycle of imbalance, contributing to poor health.

How Much Sleep Should I Get?

Before creating a perfect sleep routine, the last thing to keep in mind is how much sleep you should actually be getting. Remember the sleep cycles discussed in the last chapter? Each night, the body needs to go through several rounds of this cycle, each one lasting around 90 minutes. It's recommended to get at least four but up to six sleep cycles per night. Adults should then aim to get seven hours of sleep at night at the very least, though up to nine can also be beneficial.

Everyone's body is different, so only you can determine how much sleep works best for you. Start with eight hours, and if you find that you have a busy schedule, see if you can reduce it to seven. If you find that eight is not enough, try getting nine and notice how you might feel based on different schedules.

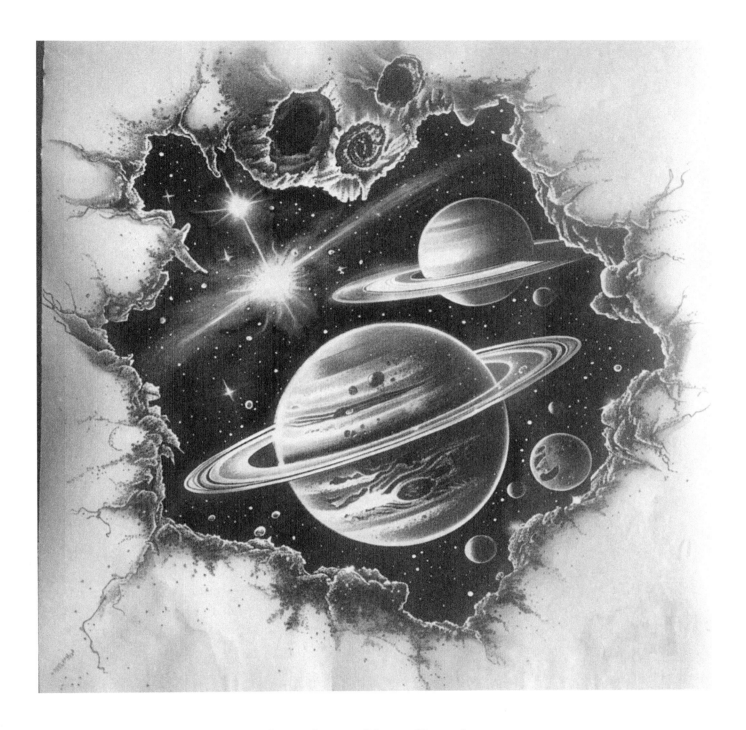

Creating a Sleep Routine

Creating a solid sleep routine isn't just about going to sleep and waking up at the same time. The things we do throughout the day, before bed, and after we wake up can all impact our quality of sleep. By allowing your tasks, habits, and daily demands to fall within a structured schedule, it becomes easier to maintain a routine that promotes total health.

Organizing your day is a powerful way to reduce stress and feelings of overwhelm. Below is a guide to help you understand the important elements of your routine, allowing you to build a schedule that aligns with your basic needs.

Routine Element	Tips and Guidance
Wake Time	When you wake up in the morning depends on your schedule. One important consideration to make is sleep inertia. Upon waking, we often feel tired and groggy as our minds adjust. This period can last for as little as 15 minutes or as long as an hour (Pacheco, 2024a). Give yourself at least an hour to get ready in the morning so you aren't expected to dive into work right away. For example, if you have to clock in at 9:00 a.m., don't expect to roll out of bed at 8:30 and rush out the door. Give your mind and body time to adjust, as well as extra time to do some of the things mentioned next, and you will find that you become more productive. Maintain a regular wake time each morning to help with body regulation and consistency.
Morning Light Exposure	Research shows that exposure to natural light during the day helps regulate our body's internal clock, promoting better night-time sleep, and could even have antidepressant effects (Blume, 2019). If you take the time to expose yourself to natural light in the morning, you promote wakefulness and give your body a vital signal that it's time to wake up—and you may find yourself becoming more alert. In the winter months, a bright light box can help with waking up and managing your circadian rhythm. These are lights specifically made to induce alertness and treat sleep conditions. Direct the beam of light toward you during morning activities to provide a slight energy boost and regulate your circadian rhythm. Enjoy your morning coffee or tea outside and let the sunshine on your face. Open the curtains when you wake up, and consider going on a morning walk. Adding an element of natural light exposure to your daily routine in the morning can have many benefits.
Morning Physical Activity	As mentioned, cortisol is released in the morning, providing you with a feeling of alertness. This gives you a boost of energy, perfect for adding in some morning physical activity. This can help reduce stress and anxiety, and aid in hormonal regulation. You'll also feel accomplished and confident to face the day after completing a quick workout in the morning! At the end of the chapter, you'll find specific types of physical activity to try.

Morning Ritual	It can be helpful to introduce a morning ritual to aid in mood regulation. Consider something like journaling, which allows you to get your thoughts out and reduce stress first thing in the morning. Doing breathwork can also help regulate your system for the rest of the day. More holistic tips will be discussed later in the book, but it's important to consider some of these approaches now so you can start thinking about creating your own morning ritual. This gives you something to look forward to and helps you start your day off in a positive way. If you give yourself plenty of time to wake up and adjust each morning, you might find you're more productive and efficient, versus rushing out the door last minute for work.
First Meal	Since our metabolism relies so heavily on hormones and sleep, you might be wondering when is the best time to have your first meal. According to some experts, it's important to eat within an hour of waking up ("The Best," 2023). This can provide your body with energy and kickstart your metabolism for better digestion. Skipping breakfast could lead to excessive hunger, which may stress the body. However, this can vary between people, so it is best to observe your own body's response.
Caffeine Cut Off	Limit caffeine intake after a certain point in your schedule, as it can interfere with falling asleep later on. According to Matthew Walker, a professor of neuroscience and psychology at the University of California, Berkeley, and founder and director of the Center for Human Sleep Science, the average quarter-life of caffeine is 12 hours (Walker, n.d.). This means that 12 hours after caffeine consumption, a quarter of that caffeine is still circulating in the body! Even though you might still be able to fall asleep after your cola with dinner or coffee with dessert, it could disrupt how much deep sleep you're able to get. If possible, cut off caffeine 12 hours before bed—meaning that if you want to fall asleep by 11:00 p.m., don't have any after 11:00 a.m. Switch to caffeine-free drinks, and consider lower-caffeine alternatives for the morning, such as green tea over coffee. If you find you become sleepy throughout the day, consider trying to hydrate more with water or a hydrating fruit like an apple. This could boost your energy, helping you finish up work so you can get to sleep at a decent time.

Last Meal	Avoid heavy meals close to bedtime that might cause discomfort or indigestion during the night. Certain sleep positions can cause heartburn or digestion issues, leading to upset stomachs in the morning or having to get up to go to the bathroom in the middle of the night. To promote better digestion, it's best to sleep on your left side and with your head elevated and avoid sleeping on your stomach (Chesak, 2023). Food also provides your body with energy, so meals too close to bed could cause unnecessary alertness. A good rule to follow is to stop eating three hours before bed (Peters, 2023).
Nightly Physical Activity	For some people's schedules, the best time to work out might be later at night. However, if exercise happens too late or close to bedtime, this can affect your sleep due to increased adrenaline levels. Adrenaline, like cortisol, helps keep the body alert, which is needed for exercise. When exercising at night, choose something a little less strenuous, like stretching. However, even during lighter exercise, insulin sensitivity is enhanced (Everett, 2013). Insulin sensitivity refers to the body's ability to manage blood sugar, an important element of sleep health. When the muscles use up blood sugar during contractions induced by exercise, glucose is controlled. This is important as research shows higher blood sugar levels are correlated with poorer sleep quality (Pacheco, 2023). In addition, less intense exercise that doesn't increase adrenaline has been proven to improve sleep quality and strengthen "the relaxation response" (DiNardo, 2020).
Last Hydration	Limit fluid intake close to bedtime if nighttime urination is disrupting your sleep. The body can process liquids in as little as five minutes (Tinsley, 2023); however, it may take longer depending on the amount and other factors. Avoid drinking excessive amounts of water within an hour before bed, taking only small sips to curb thirst until then.
Blue Light Cut Off	As mentioned previously, light can drastically disrupt your sleep. For this reason, avoid screens for at least an hour before bedtime to limit exposure to blue light. Blue light is the light emitted by electronics like phones, tablets, and TV screens. This light simulates sunlight, making our bodies feel more alert, and impacting our circadian rhythm and hormones in the process. It's essential to reduce phone use before bed to prevent the suprachiasmatic nucleus from releasing cortisol due to the "blue wavelength light from LED-based devices" (Rosen, 2015). In addition, blue light blocks the release of melatonin (Salamon, 2022). If you do have to use a screen, such as for shift work close to nighttime,

	consider using a blue light blocker on the computer that automatically comes on, like f.lux. This is also good as it can remind you it's time to turn off the screen soon. If using your phone, take advantage of night mode to change the screen. Avoid using mobile phones too close to bedtime, and keep them away from where you sleep to avoid temptation. Instead, consider reading or doing a low-pressure craft, such as knitting, to keep your mind busy while your body prepares for sleep.
Wind Down Time	Just like creating a morning ritual, it's also important to consider introducing a nightly routine that will help you wind down before bed. Consider something like listening to an audiobook or podcast that isn't too exciting. In addition, use an auto-timer to stop after 15 minutes or so. This is long enough to listen to something to stop overthinking, but it's also not too exciting to keep you up for the next chapter! Consider fiction as the content may be more "low stakes" and avoids getting into thinking or problem-solving mode from nonfiction. It's important to have a ritual to finish the day so your mind isn't busy thinking about the stressors of yesterday and the fears of tomorrow.
Reducing Nightly Stress	Whatever you do, ensure you plan ahead so something doesn't come to your mind later that night causing you to stay up another couple of hours to complete the task. Use positive visualization about the next day to set you up for success. If you think to yourself, *I really can't do all the work I have to do tomorrow; it's so overwhelming,* this causes stress at night, disrupting your sleep and making it hard to work the next day. If, instead, you say, *I got this! Tomorrow might be busy, but I know I'll get it all done,* it can help induce a more positive and uplifting mindset. Positive visualization will ensure you stop overthinking and feel more motivated the next day.

Reduce stress in holistic ways by using things like breathwork, journaling, and hot baths before bed (see Chapter 5 for more details). Try listening to calming music or nature sounds before bed as part of your relaxation routine. Instead of boosting cortisol, facilitate an environment that regulates your hormones before bed, thus inducing deeper sleep. |
| **Sleep Time** | Just like waking up, pick a time that you can consistently get to sleep every night. Make sure your nightly routine starts before the actual time you want to fall asleep. For example, perhaps you have to wake by 7:00 a.m. to have time to exercise, make breakfast, and get ready for work. This would mean you would need to be asleep by 12:00 a.m. at the latest. In this situation, you would want to be in bed, under the covers, and ready to fall asleep by 11:40 p.m., as it takes 15-20 minutes to fall asleep (Rausch-Phung & Rehman, 2023). Try to give yourself an hour to fall asleep because if you manage to fall asleep in just 10 minutes, you give yourself even more sleep time. |

Aim to maintain a consistent sleep schedule, even on weekends. Weekends are often thought to be opportunities to catch up on sleep, but if you maintain a healthy sleep routine throughout the week, you won't need to catch up! Use the extra time in the morning to catch up on personal passions and projects, and create more relaxation rather than spending your mornings sleeping in. Schedule a nap on the weekends as you're figuring out your sleep schedule regularity if you need to catch up. For more nap tips, see Chapter 5!

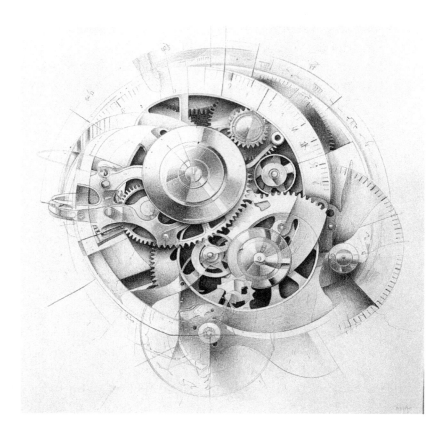

Your Routine Template

Now that you've taken the time to understand the elements of your routine, you can craft your own ideal sleep schedule. Below is an empty template for you to use to help ensure you have the perfect day for facilitating healthy sleep.

The first column includes the routine element we discussed. The column in the middle is for you to write down the time you intend to do this, helping you plan ahead. Then, the last column provides a spot for you to include any to-dos or notes. For example, for wake time, you might write down that you are going to shower or take the dog outside first thing. In the caffeine cut-off box, you might write a reminder to sip on some herbal tea or fill up your water bottle to promote hydration. You can copy this template and use it daily to write in meals and other important reminders for daily consistency.

Routine Element	Time	Tasks or Notes
Wake Time	__:__	
Morning Light Exposure	__:__	
Morning Physical Activity	__:__	
Morning Ritual	__:__	
First Meal	__:__	
Caffeine Cut-Off	__:__	
Last Meal	__:__	

Nightly Physical Activity	__:__	
Last Hydration	__:__	
Blue Light Cut-Off	__:__	
Wind-Down Time	__:__	
Reducing Nightly Stress	__:__	
Sleep Time	__:__	

Take Action During the Day

There are many things you can do during the day to promote better sleep at night. Below are a few additional tools and tips to help you make the most of your daily routine.

Sleep and Food Tracking Template

To identify issues that may be affecting your sleep quality, using a sleep and food tracking template can uncover patterns so you can troubleshoot issues. Below is a template that tracks how you feel throughout the day, enabling you to make correlations between habits and health.

Date:_____	Time Period	Feelings (Physical)	Feelings (Emotional)
When I Woke Up			
How Long It Took to Wake Up			
What I Ate and Drank for Breakfast			
Morning Stressors			

What I Ate and Drank for Lunch			
Afternoon Stressors			
What I Ate and Drank for Dinner			
Nightly Stressors			
How Long It Took to Fall Asleep			
What Time I Fell Asleep			

Physical Activity Guide

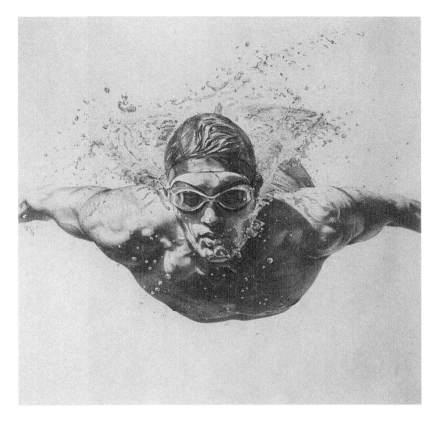

Different types of exercise might have a different impact on the body. Below are a few exercises to consider based on when they should ideally be performed. The impact they have, their intensity, and the energy required differ for various exercises, so incorporate them into your day at the right time for the best results!

For Morning Exercises	For Nightly Exercise
• walking/running • swimming • pilates • strength training	• yoga (low-impact moves) • walking (slow pace) • resistance exercises (using no weights) • progressive muscle relaxation
Exercise in the morning is a great way to get your blood pumping and kickstart your energy for the day. Choose exercises that make you feel alert and ready to take on the day!	The important thing to remember about nightly exercise is that it should be slow and intuitive. Focus on breathing and relaxation and release from stretches and movements rather than pushing yourself too hard.

Chapter 3:

Staying Asleep—Managing What Keeps

You Awake

Once you have the perfect routine and are taking the right steps to get rested before bed, it's then important to figure out what foods, habits, and other things in your life are keeping you awake throughout the night.

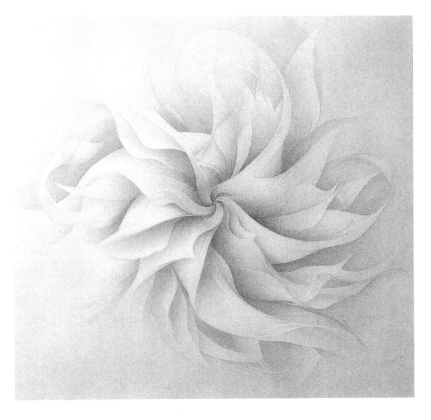

Whole Health Sleep

Knowing the science behind sleep is an important foundation for getting deeper rest, but beyond this, it's a good idea to look at some of the more practical aspects of daily life that might impede your sleep.

How Does My Diet Impact Sleep?

Everything we put into our body goes through our digestive system, which works hard to filter through the various things we provide. Because of this, everything we consume can have an impact on the body. The vitamins and minerals we provide, or fail to provide, are responsible for nourishing us from the inside out. In addition, what we eat impacts our health throughout the day. If you aren't providing your body with enough nutrients, you may have other symptoms that impact your hormones.

There isn't always a clear correlation between what we consume and how we sleep (such as how caffeine might induce quicker alertness). Hence, it's important to consider how the things we put in our bodies might be contributing to various aspects of our health.

What Foods Are the Worst for Sleep?

While it's important to not demonize certain foods, it is equally crucial to consider how our diet might be causing negative sleep patterns. Spicy, fatty, and sugary foods are the worst for sleep, as well as anything caffeinated. As mentioned previously, it's important to cut yourself off from caffeine after a certain point to reduce wakefulness close to bed.

Sugary and fatty foods could also cause energy spikes due to increased blood sugar. If you do find you indulge, try doing some light stretches to use up some of that blood sugar and induce sleepiness. Spicy foods or big meals can also disrupt your digestion due to indigestion or heartburn, so limit these before bed as well.

What Foods Are the Best for Better Sleep?

Foods better for sleep have a few components that induce better energy regulation and wakefulness, such as:

- **Magnesium**: An increase in magnesium has been found to help with sleep (Wilson, 2018). Choose foods like leafy greens. For more on magnesium, check out the appendix for further reading.

- **Melatonin**: Foods high in melatonin help promote sleepiness. Pistachios contain melatonin, making them a useful nighttime snack.

- **Tryptophan**: Tryptophan is good for regulating your mood and helps with serotonin and melatonin production in the body, both essential hormones for sleep management (Summer, 2024a). Lean meats, like chicken, turkey, and fish are high in tryptophan. See the chart toward the end of this chapter to discover more sleep-promoting foods!

- **Carbohydrates**: Carbohydrate-rich foods can increase "the uptake of tryptophan by the brain (Benton, 2022)." Just ensure they are carbohydrates that are low-to-medium on the glycemic index to avoid spikes and crashes in blood sugar. For more on blood glucose and brain health, see the appendix for further reading.

These are just a few elements to consider when choosing snacks or meals close to bed. Below you'll find a more detailed chart of what foods to eat and what should be avoided.

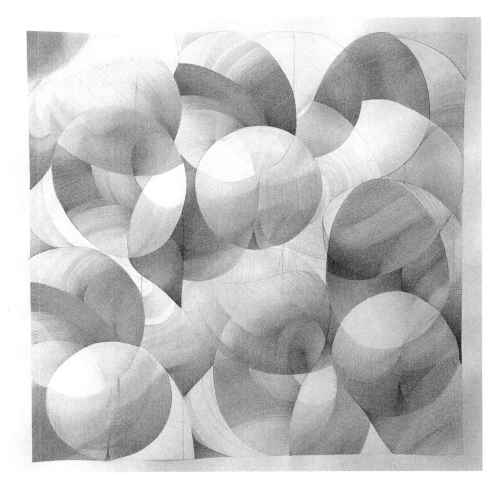

Why Is It So Hard to Wake Up in the Morning?

Trouble waking in the morning can mess up your routine, so you might be wondering why it's so difficult for you to wake up and emerge from bed. Oversleeping is easy for some to do, and the snooze button on alarms makes that even easier! First, it's important to determine if you are getting deep, restful sleep each night. If you are not, you might find that your body craves more sleep, thus making it harder to get up in the morning.

Next, consider if there are any habits that make it difficult to get out of bed, such as staying up too late on electronic devices. For example, if you find yourself using social media while in bed, you may discover that you attempt to sleep later to make up for lost time at night. In addition, if you have a schedule that forces you to start work right away, it can be hard for your tired and vulnerable mind to find the motivation to begin, thus sleeping in later as a form of procrastination.

Aside from habits, there could be something physical going on in your body, such as a hormonal balance or a type of food that keeps you from getting a restful night's sleep. It's not always about what we do in the morning but rather what's going on at night that can make it challenging to get out of bed.

What Causes Insomnia?

Sometimes, the biggest disturbances are sleep disorders, such as insomnia. Insomnia may be caused by many different things, such as (Suni, 2024c):

- physiological arousal at unwanted times

- family history

- age and gender

- mental health disorders

- increased cortisol

Insomnia is characterized by ("Insomnia," n.d.):
- trouble falling asleep

- difficulty staying asleep

- daytime sleepiness

One helpful method of managing insomnia is through the use of cognitive behavioral therapy (CBT). CBT emphasizes how thoughts and behavior correlate, with a focus on restructuring mental habits for more favorable outcomes. This evidence-based approach is aimed at reducing disruptive thoughts and inducing more mindfulness. Some CBT-based techniques to help with insomnia include:

- meditation

- breathing exercises

- progressive muscle relaxation

You can find more about how to start these practices in the appendix, or by clicking here! If after the implementation of these practices, you don't start to see improvements in insomnia and sleep health, it's important to see a professional to rule out potential underlying conditions that induce insomnia (Newsom, 2024b).

Troubleshooting Sleep Disturbances

Remember that it's not just the quantity and quality of your sleep that matters—aim for uninterrupted deep sleep cycles. Below are some tips for overcoming the biggest sleep disturbances you may be facing.

Sleep Health and Others

It's not always what's going on in your body that is impacting your sleep but the disrupting factors around you, such as kids and pets. Use these tips to help tackle the things that might be keeping you awake at night.

Pets	<ul><li>Pets operate on different circadian rhythms than humans, especially felines as they are crepuscular and most active at dawn and dusk ("Cat," n.d.). For this reason, do your best to avoid keeping your pet in the room with you.</li><li>At first, it might be hard as you may enjoy falling asleep with them around, or they may miss you at night and cause disruptions by scratching or whining at the door.</li><li>To make the transition easier, ensure they get enough physical activity during the day by playing with them or taking them on a walk. This can help ensure they are more likely to sleep at night.</li><li>If you are unable to separate them from your sleeping environment, encourage them to at least sleep on the floor rather than your bed so you do not wake from their movement throughout the night.</li></ul>
Kids	<ul><li>Children need strong routines for proper development. If your child wakes you up throughout the night, it's important to practice establishing stronger bedtime routines that match yours to encourage them to stay asleep if you are cosleeping. If you are transitioning from or wanting to avoid cosleeping, then establishing strong bedtime rituals can help.</li><li>Use the same tips throughout the book to help your child get better sleep just as you use for yourself, such as the environmental factors for their bedroom in the upcoming Chapter 4.</li></ul>

	• Just as you do with your pets, ensure your children are getting enough physical activity throughout the day to encourage them to sleep more heavily throughout the night, and pick nutrient-rich foods over sugary sweets to avoid energy spikes.
	• Practice and patience are key as you establish a routine. It may take some time to fully adjust, but with important boundaries and rituals, your child will find a healthy sleep pattern.
Restless or Snoring Partners	• Partners who toss and turn at night can be disruptive for those they share a bed with, especially if the other person is a light sleeper. Use the tips throughout the book with your partner so they can find help just as you are!
	• Invite them to join you on a nightly walk, or spend some time before bed decompressing with them and talking about your thoughts and feelings. You may find that they are restless at night due to emotional reasons, so sharing your feelings is a great way to connect to each other and work through disturbances.
	• If they continue to disrupt your sleep, it may be time to encourage them to seek professional help. A sleep study could troubleshoot issues that are keeping them awake throughout the night.
	• When all else fails, consider separate beds. You can use two twin beds pushed together, or a separate room if your partner struggles with snoring. Snoring can often be a sign that something else is going on, like sleep apnea, so if snoring is this disruptive, encourage them to seek professional assessments to rule out underlying conditions. If you don't want to use separate beds, at least using separate sheets and blankets on top of the bed can help prevent disturbances.
Differing Schedules	• If you and your partner have different schedules, such as one working night shifts and the other working in the morning, this may disturb both of your sleep routines.
	• To start, lay out clothes the night before so one partner doesn't disturb the other by digging through drawers and closets. Have meals prepped and everything ready before sleep times to ensure no partner is woken up by other noises in the house.
	• Use sleep masks and noise machines to drown out sound and light that

the other partner might have to use when getting ready in the morning.

- Use a nightlight or adjustable light bulb to keep bathrooms and hallways outside of the bedroom more softly lit to reduce disturbances.

Stress Reminders

Occasional sleep disturbances might not have serious underlying causes and could simply be temporary. Avoid getting overly worried about waking up in the middle of the night if it happens on occasion, or during the initial stages while you're still working on your sleep. When you find yourself waking up in the middle of the night, stop the panic! That will only alert your brain more by causing unnecessary stress. Everyone has an occasional restless night—don't let one bad night lead to anxiety about not sleeping well in the future.

Below are some tips to help you reduce stress and worry over sleep disturbances:

- Avoid clock-watching as this can increase stress levels when trying to fall asleep. If you were supposed to be asleep by 10:00 p.m. and midnight is approaching, that's okay! You may have one night of poor sleep, but don't let this disrupt your entire schedule.

- If you wake up in the middle of the night, resist the urge to check your phone. The light can stimulate wakefulness. While you might want to check social media to distract yourself from stress, chances are it will only make it worse and delay your ability to fall asleep.

- Don't lie awake in bed if you can't fall asleep within 20 minutes. Get up and do something relaxing until you feel sleepy again. Laying there and panicking might induce more worry, so getting out of bed and distracting yourself with something (other than your phone) can help. Consider something productive and light, such as folding a load of laundry or laying out your outfit for the next day.

- Use positive visualization and affirmations to help you stop the worry and prepare for the day ahead. Small moments of reassurance will induce relaxation and focus so you can overcome your most panicked thoughts. Positive reminders might include phrases such as:

  o I am fine, and I will feel fine tomorrow.

  o It's okay to miss a little sleep. I'm just feeling nervous about tomorrow but will be fine by the end of the day.

  o I don't need to focus on anything right now other than relaxing.

- My mind is wandering, but that's normal at this time of night. My anxiety will soon pass.

- Don't change your schedule due to a restless night. Stay on track and remind yourself it'll all be fine soon. It's better to have one restless night and move past it quickly than it is to disrupt your entire week trying to make up for one night of missed sleep.

Common Stimulants

The biggest stimulants that may be keeping you up at night are alcohol, caffeine, and nicotine.

Alcohol	Caffeine	Nicotine
Alcohol may make you feel drowsy initially, but it can disrupt your sleep later in the night. The more you drink, the more likely you are to notice sleep disturbances. Limit drinking at least three hours before bed (Bryan, 2024c).	Caffeine might mask sleepiness and provide a feeling of alertness, but in reality, all it does is block adenosine (Pacheco, 2024b). It's best to avoid caffeine at least 8 hours before bed, but preferably 12.	Smoking, chewing, and vaping tobacco are all detrimental forms of nicotine consumption that have a myriad of negative health impacts, one of them being poor sleep. Smokers are 50% more likely to have sleep disturbances (Newsom, 2023). Avoid using nicotine altogether, but especially four hours before bed.

Sleep-Focused Food Guide

To Eat	Sleep Benefits
Chamomile	<ul><li>This herb is known for having mild tranquilizing properties, as well as reducing stress-inducing hormones (Gupta, 2010).</li><li>Drink chamomile tea before bed to feel the benefits of this powerful natural remedy (just make sure to sip small amounts earlier in the evening to avoid waking up for urination throughout the night).</li></ul>

Kiwi	• Studies show kiwi consumption can help induce better quality sleep (Suni, 2024b). • Eat kiwi one hour before bed to employ the antioxidant properties of this fuzzy fruit.
Lean Protein	• Many types of lean proteins include tryptophan, which is important for creating serotonin and melatonin in the brain (Sheikh, 2023). • Choose plant-based proteins like legumes or tofu for your last meal of the day.
Nuts/Seeds	• Many nuts and seeds are magnesium-rich, helpful for inducing sleepiness and regulating cognitive functions throughout the day. • Choose nuts like almonds, walnuts, and pistachios (Suni, 2024b).
Leafy Greens	• Many leafy greens are rich in magnesium, like kale and spinach. • They also contain calcium, which helps reduce stress and stabilize the brain ("Foods", 2020).

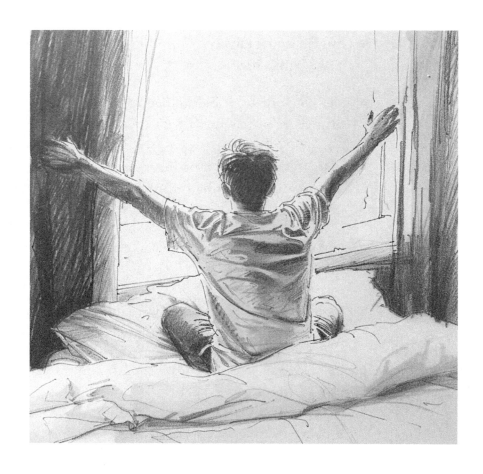

Get Up and Stay Up

Not everyone is a morning person! In fact, some research suggests as few as 15% of people are "morning larks" (Martin, 2023). However, don't fret! There are things you can do that will make it easier for you to wake up in the morning feeling rested and ready for the day ahead. This includes things like:

1. **Make your alarm clock inaccessible** so you have to actually get up to turn it off. If you use your phone, plug it into a charger across the room. Better yet, put it in the bathroom if you have one connected to your bedroom, just keep the door open to ensure you hear it. This will give your brain a little more time to adjust to waking up, potentially inducing more logical thinking that will keep you from crawling back into bed!

2. **Get a head start on the day** by laying out your clothes and having a yummy (low-sugar) breakfast or coffee ready to go. When you reduce the amount of work you have to do *and* create something to look forward to, you can start the day off on a positive note.

3. **Start with physical movement**. Lay out your shoes the night before so you can look forward to your morning walk. Have a warm towel or comfy bathrobe waiting for you after the workout so you can enjoy a hot shower.

4. **Do something you enjoy** before diving into work or schoolwork for the day, such as reading a novel, writing in a journal, or doing something artistic, like drawing. This can help your brain slowly adjust and keep a lighthearted tone at the beginning of your day.

One or a combination of these things can make it easier for you to wake up, even if you don't consider yourself a morning person now! The more you wake up at a certain time, the easier it becomes to adjust, so don't give up hope if you don't feel alert right away in the morning. After a few weeks, you will find yourself more naturally waking up at this time.

Chapter 4:

Environmental Factors

—Creating the Perfect Sleep Situation

It's not just our schedule that impacts sleep, but also our surroundings—whether that's our mattress or our mindset.

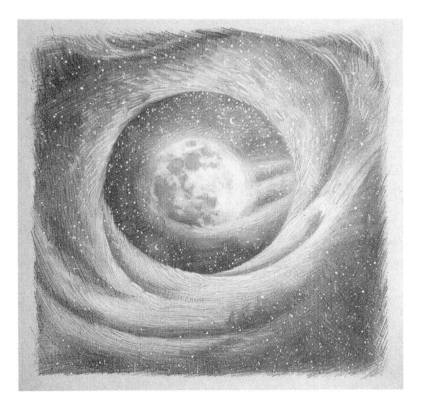

The Impact of Our Surroundings

It's human nature to maintain awareness of our surroundings, at least on some level. Consider how you may notice a snake crossing your path during a nature walk. We are inclined to give a certain amount of energy to our surroundings to ensure we stay safe. It's a survival system naturally wired into our bodies.

Because of this, however, our surroundings can sometimes have a big impact on how we sleep. From temperature to clutter, there are many ways our surroundings can affect our sleep.

How Does Temperature Impact Sleep?

Throughout the day, our bodies adjust temperatures based on the exposure to sun we feel. A few hours before falling asleep, our body temperature starts to drop and continues to do so until the morning, when it rises again. During the day, body temperature typically remains around 98.6 °F (or 37 °C) (Pacheco, 2024c).

For this reason, it's helpful to sleep in a cooler environment to support melatonin's efforts and remind your brain that it's time to sleep. Just like you would want to turn the lights off to simulate the feeling of night, use cooler temperatures in your bedroom for the same effect.

What Sounds Can Keep Me Awake?

Any noise you hear is one that has the potential to disturb deep sleep, even if it doesn't wake you up all the way. Have you ever tried to avoid disturbing someone sleeping, only for a noise you make to cause them to stir? They might have remained asleep, but they still heard the noise, and there's a chance it disrupted their sleep cycles.

Noise disturbances at night might increase adrenaline or cortisol. Some research also suggests we may be even more sensitive to noise at night than when awake, so it's crucial to take extra care to reduce noise for better sleep (Summer, 2024d).

From noisy neighbors to sleeping partners, there's a lot that could be keeping you awake. It's best to avoid any noise, if possible, when you are sleeping. Try to first remedy these noise disturbances, and then if you can't, utilize methods to reduce the noise. This could mean using earplugs or a noise machine to drown out other sounds.

What Should I Wear to Bed?

Clothes impact sleep because they regulate our temperature and provide comfort. When choosing clothes to wear to bed, start by picking loose-fitting pajamas. If they are too tight or compressive, it may prevent your body from being able to fully relax.

Loose clothes are also better as they allow your skin to breathe, providing more regulation of your body temperature. Clothes that are too thick and tight could make you feel hot and restricted.

Pick clothes in layers as well. Rather than wearing a sweatshirt and sweatpants to bed, you might choose instead to wear a light T-shirt and shorts, with a sweater or extra blanket. This way, if you wake up and are too hot at night, you can easily take off a layer without disturbing your sleep.

Does a Cluttered Bedroom Impact My Sleep Health?

Since we are so aware of our surroundings, that means every little thing in our environment is something that has the potential to take our attention. If you find yourself struggling to fall asleep at night and stress becomes the norm, it might be due to the clutter in your surroundings.

A cluttered space might show that something is going on negatively with your overall mental health and well-being (Carollo, 2024). It's important to work on reducing clutter and maintaining an organized space to promote better sleep overall.

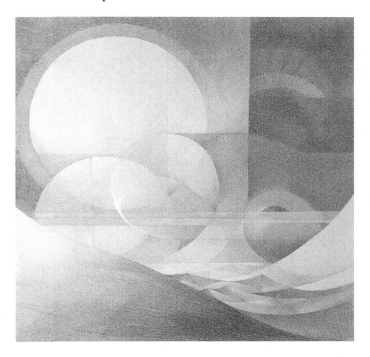

Perfecting Your Sleep Environment

As you start to manage your hormones, diet, and routine, you will start to notice changes in your sleep health. But to make things even better, and to promote consistency, it's also important to perfect your sleep environment.

De-Cluttering For Sleep

Below are some tips to help you create a harmonious situation that allows you to balance sleep and overall health:

- **Make your bedroom a sleep-specific space**: Keep work-related activities out of the bedroom. This space should be associated only with relaxation. This means moving your home office or video game setup elsewhere when possible. These will serve as reminders of work or stressors, which could make it difficult to reduce alertness at night.

- **Hide away clutter**: Even if you can't get rid of all of your clutter, or if it will take a longer time to clean up your space, start by at least removing it from the bedroom. If it is out of your sight, it will be easier to reduce the impact it may have on your ability to fall asleep.

- **Remove surfaces that promote clutter**: If you have a large end table or chair in the corner, you might find it collects clutter or extra clothing. Remove anything that seems to collect a lot of excessive stuff, and consider a more minimalist aesthetic for a better sleep space.

- **Use an area rug for hard floors and thick curtains for windows**: These will add a sense of warmth and comfort, while also serving as additional sound-proofing measures.

- **Keep a trash bin in the bedroom**: This way, you can remove any additional clutter easily without having to fully leave the bedroom, enabling you to quickly clean up before bed each night.

- **Pick warm colors and monochromatic themes**: Save exciting decor for outside the bedroom and keep things cool and collected around the area where you sleep. Pick shades of tan, brown, orange, and yellow to make your space homey and under-stimulating.

- **Avoid decorative elements**: Things like bedside trinkets or decorative pieces throughout the bedroom take up space and contribute to feelings of clutter. Less is more in the bedroom to help promote sleep and relaxation.

Ideal Sleeping Conditions

Below is a quick guide to use to help you formulate the best sleep situations for better rest.

Environmental Element	Ideal Situation	Tips	Alternatives
Temperature	• 65–68 °F (18–20 °C) (Pacheco, 2024c).	• Use an area fan to keep the room cool while doubling as a sound machine. • Set your thermostat to automatically drop the temperature at night and increase it in the morning.	• Take a cool shower at night to help your body temperature decrease, especially in the summer.

Light	• Complete darkness.	• Use an eye mask to help block out any light, both natural and artificial. • Use blackout curtains in the bedroom to ensure no light slips in.	• Use a timed night light if you find it difficult to fall asleep in pitch black. This way, it will turn off a little while after you fall asleep.
Sound	• No sound at all.	• Use earplugs to help reduce noise heard from outside or partners. • Invest in sound panels to help reduce noise from downstairs, upstairs, and next-door neighbors that are keeping you awake throughout the night.	• If you find earplugs make it difficult to sleep comfortably or use your alarm, consider using a noise machine. • Choose natural sounds like running water or rain to avoid anything that might keep you alert.
Comfort	• The ideal sleep position is on your side or back (Suni, 2024a).	• Whether you like a firm or soft mattress is based on your body and preferences, such as your weight, height, and position to sleep in. Choose one that is a supportive, level mattress with a moderately thick pillow.	• Use a knee pillow for more comfortable sleeping. This can help take some tension off of your hips if you are a side sleeper.

Screen Detox

Modern life has a big impact on our sleep health. One of the biggest factors that keeps you awake at night is likely technology. Technology is not all bad, and many people need it for their work. However, excessive social media use can have an impact on our health.

One survey showed over 90% of smartphone users used their device at bedtime (Alshobaili, 2019). This is a prevalent issue that keeps many people from getting the rest they need. Below are some tips to help you try a screen detox:

- Pick a day out of the week to **completely shut off from your phone**. Only answer emergency calls, and ignore all texts, notifications, and emails. Utilize non-screen activities to help you get used to the avoidance of your phone, and write down how you feel throughout the day to stay aware of the sensations you have.

- Make a rule to **keep your phone out of the bedroom**. Invest in an alarm clock to wake you up in the morning instead of your phone. Schedule an hour or so well before bed to check in with any social media to help you resist the urge later on.

- **Set time limits on various apps** to prevent overusing them, and consider changing your phone to all black and white to make it less exciting. Our phones provide instant gratification, so anything we do to reduce their appeal is helpful in reducing impulsivity and overuse.

Chapter 5:

Boosting Restfulness—Holistic

Approaches

for Long-Term Health

When we can't sleep, it's tempting to reach for extra-strong, highly caffeinated drinks to keep you awake. But instead of relying on short-term solutions, take holistic approaches for better health.

There's not one quick fix to get better sleep. Instead, the focus should be on incorporating small habits over time that will contribute to an overall better routine.

Natural remedies and holistic approaches are always a first suggestion to remedy sleep as they are accessible, more likely to be risk-free, and work with your body's natural processes to facilitate improvement. Below, you will find two categories: restfulness tools and relaxation strategies.

Restfulness tools might cost a little more money, but they don't necessarily have to be expensive. These are tools to add to your toolbox of sleep health for improvement. The second category, relaxation strategies, are mostly costless suggestions, but they're very valuable in the help they can add to your sleep routine. Try each one to see if it makes an impact, and create a strategy that works for your personal needs.

These additions to your sleep routine are not guaranteed to help, but they are approaches that could positively impact your overall health. Experiment with one or two a week to help build up your routine over time.

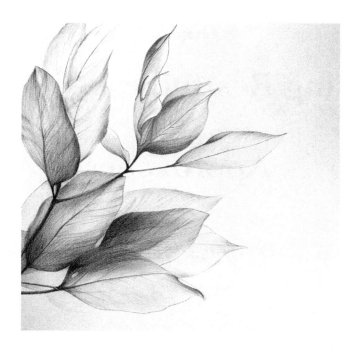

Restfulness Tools

Below are a few restful tools to consider adding into your daily or weekly routine. They may take longer to have a positive impact, but with patience and dedication, they are sure to create a solid routine.

Teas

Herbal tea is a great way to add more natural remedies to your routine. Warm tea provides a sense of peace and restfulness when you're winding down at night. Sip tea when journaling during the evening or while enjoying some time outside under the moonlight. The best teas for better sleep health are:

- Lavender
- Chamomile
- Mint

Essential Oils

Certain essential oils might contain compounds that can promote restfulness and improve sleep health. Consider trying some of the ones that promote better sleep below (Wong, 2023):

- Bergamot
- Cedarwood
- Lavender

Essential oils can be added to a warm bath or used in an air diffuser for aromatherapy. Some, as long as they are safe to do so, can be dabbed on your skin or added to body lotion to promote more restfulness.

Supplements

Taking a certain vitamin, mineral, or other dietary supplement in pill form is an easy and accessible method of adding this desired chemical to your body on a consistent basis. The best supplements for sleep health are:

- Magnesium

- Melatonin

- L-theanine

Be sure to check with your doctor when taking other medications, or if you've been diagnosed with a condition that might interact with various supplements.

Weighted Blanket

A weighted blanket is like a normal blanket, but it is often filled with weights to provide more pressure. You can make a homemade weighted blanket by following one of many free tutorials online, or you can purchase one for your bed.

A weighted blanket will apply pressure across your body, which can provide you with a sense of comfort. When you feel comforted and relaxed, you are less likely to tense your muscles, thus leaving you more satisfied and able to get better rest.

Mouth Guard

If you find that you grind your teeth at night, a mouth guard is a great addition for those who want better sleep. This will help prevent your jaw from tensing as much, alleviating some jaw and tooth pain in the process. Check with your dentist to see if they recommend a specific mouth guard.

Regular Massages

Regular massages help relax your body and release tension that you may be holding onto. This will make you feel better, thus inducing serotonin production, which can aid with melatonin release. You can invest in a massage gun at home for personal use, or consider splurging on professional massages for even more relaxation.

Relaxation Strategies

Getting better sleep doesn't have to be expensive! For more methods of improving sleep, consider the strategies below.

Hot Baths

Baths, much like massages, offer whole-body relaxation. The warm temperature might seem counterintuitive at first since your body temperature decreases at night, but as you leave the bath, you will find you are overcome with a burst of cold! The combination of the relaxation followed by a temperature drop induces sleepiness. Add essential oils and sip herbal tea to level up your bath, and consider using a weighted blanket after you're out. As you can see, there are many ways to combine multiple strategies and tools for better sleep.

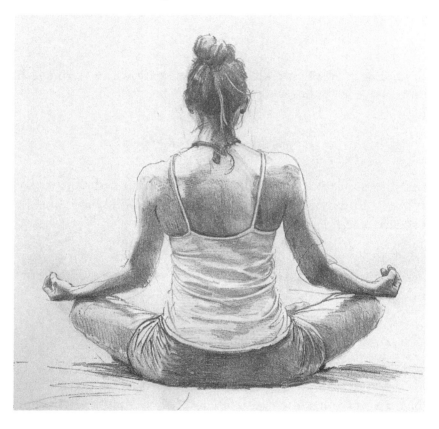

Breathwork

Many people find themselves stuck in fight-or-flight mode. This refers to the stress response triggered by a plethora of stressors throughout the day. When in fight-or-flight mode, cortisol may be released, which could mess with your sleep hormones.

Breathwork is the process of deep inhaling and exhaling in a slow and steady way to activate the parasympathetic nervous system. Doing this at night and in the morning will regulate the body and help you get out of fight/flight mode for better stress management. To practice deep breathing, follow the steps below:

1. Ensure you are in a comfortable position. Relax your shoulders, jaw, and abdomen.

2. Breathe in deeply through your nose. Don't rush the breath, but don't go so slow that you feel your lungs start to strain.

3. Hold this for a moment, and then slowly exhale. Feel as your stomach rises and falls with each breath.

4. Continue to practice this pattern of inhaling and exhaling.

5. Start with five-minute sessions and try to practice this daily, extending by a few minutes each time. Slowly extend the exhale so it becomes longer than the inhale to allow the breath to naturally pause after the exhale for a few counts before repeating the cycle. This is helpful to prevent over-breathing.

Breathwork is better supplemented by additional methods of mental relaxation, such as sleep meditation, progressive muscle relaxation, and mindfulness. To discover additional methods of mindfulness and sleep meditation, click here, or check out more books in the appendix!

Yoga Nidra

Also known as yogic sleep, this relaxation technique helps you transition from wakefulness and sleep. It's great to use for naps or when you go to bed at night. To follow the practice of Yoga Nidra, use the steps below:

1. Lie down with your eyes closed and feet elevated. If lying down is not possible, sit back in your office chair with your eyes closed.

2. Set a 30-minute alarm to ensure you wake up.

3. Use breathwork to bring awareness to your body.

4. Think of an intention, or point of visualization, that will help you focus your thoughts toward relaxation.

5. Travel through your body, focusing on different parts, one at a time.

6. Notice any sensations you have, and keep regulating your breath.

7. As your breathing starts to change, bring your focus back, and notice how different parts of your body feel as you do this.

For a guided meditation and special Yoga Nidra practice, click here, or see the additional sleep resources at the end of the book!

Napping as a Sleep Supplementation

Is napping good for you? Are naps detrimental to sleep? There is no exact yes or no answer to this question. What's important to know is how to get the right length of a nap into your routine when supplementation is necessary. Below are some tips for napping from The Sleep Foundation (Summer, 2024c):

- The ideal nap length is between 20 to 30 minutes. Anything longer might take you into deeper sleep, which requires a longer period of time. If you wake up in the middle of this deep sleep, it can make you feel even groggier than you were before the nap started.

- Avoid taking naps within eight hours of when you will go to sleep. A good rule of thumb is to cut off naps at the same time you would caffeine. Napping after lunch is a good time to take advantage of afternoon sleepiness brought on by your circadian rhythm.

- Nap in your bedroom when you can to ensure you maintain a consistent sleep environment. If you nap at your desk or workspace, you might train your mind to be more sleepy in this area. Work and sleep should be kept separate to avoid confusing the brain.

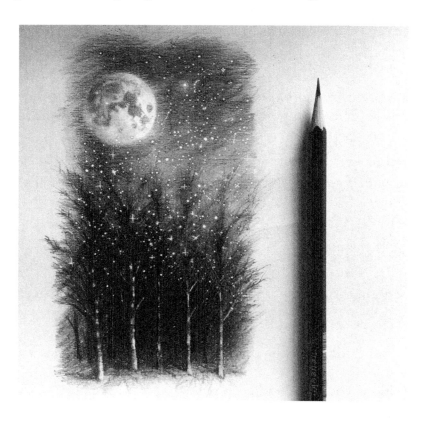

Dream Journaling

Whether you have night terrors or vivid dreams that disrupt your sleep, keeping a dream journal can help you make better sense of what's going on in your mind at night. Dreaming can be disruptive, especially if it causes you to wake up. Some night terrors may be due to REM-sleep disturbance condition, so consider seeing a healthcare professional or sleep specialist if this is a recurrent issue.

Alternatively, you may find you enjoy some of your dreams and find it difficult to wake up or transition from the dream world to the real world. Everyone dreams, even if you don't necessarily have any memory of what those dreams were. No matter what situation you are in, below are some tips to help you track your dreams and journal more frequently:

- Keep a journal by your bed, with a pen readily available so that it's easier to mark down your dreams first thing upon waking. Alternatively, use an app on your phone or your notes app to write down dreams right away. This way, you'll also have them all in one place. Keep your phone in flight mode to prevent the temptation to check social media first thing in the morning.

- Another method of dream recording to consider is a dictation app that you can use to record voice memos of your dreams. It can be faster and easier to talk about them, and you might find more comes out as you record.

- Focus on symbols first. What did you see? What location were you in? Then write down your actions—what you were doing? How you were feeling. Highlight symbols or places that seem to be common in your dreams.

- Interpret your dream using a dream dictionary to decipher symbols. What do they mean to you, and how might this be impacting your overall stress levels? This will help you in reducing and managing emotional states throughout the day.

Chapter 6:

Bonus Chapter—Sleep for Special

Circumstances

This last chapter serves as a "bonus" chapter that will provide you with tips for various special circumstances. Each section includes a quick guide to explain how this situation impacts sleep health, with a list of tips to improve things afterward. Review each category for important sleep information, or use specific strategies to treat various situations you might be dealing with.

Sleep for Kids and Teens

Why This Impacts Sleep

- **Kids:** Sleep is a restorative process for all ages, but this time at night is especially important for children as their minds are still developing. Kids may be scared to sleep alone or in the dark, further disrupting their sleep.

- **Teens:** Teens are often dealing with school stress and busy schedules that could impact their sleep. In addition, excessive access to social media and smartphones might lead them to stay up later than they should. Some research also suggests there is a shift in a teenager's biological clock, and that during adolescence, "teenagers have a natural tendency to fall asleep later and to wake up later" ("Sleep Needs," 2000).

- **Young Families:** Those with young and busy families likely have many responsibilities and different routine demands. It could be hard to maintain sleep routines due to everyone's varying schedules.

Specific Tips for Sleep

- Ensure toddlers get 11 to 14 hours of daily sleep. Children 4 to 5 years should get 10 to 13 hours a day, and 6- to 12-year-olds should sleep 9 to 12 hours daily. Teens should get 8 to 10 hours of sleep a night (Suni, 2024d).

- Every tip mentioned previously about creating structured routines and perfect sleep environments applies to people of all ages. One thing to make this easier is to create a nightly routine. Perhaps you can take turns picking out a relaxing family-friendly movie while everyone enjoys calming tea. You can tuck children into bed and read them a fun bedtime story that they get to pick out.

- Invest in a fun night light to help kids feel safe and happy in their rooms. You can also consider using softer lighting in the bathroom to help induce more sleepiness. Just ensure it isn't too dark! The combination of warmth and soft lighting will help them become sleepier.

- Have teens turn their devices over to parents at night to ensure they aren't up late. Setting rules and boundaries with technology will help them develop a stronger relationship with it into adulthood.

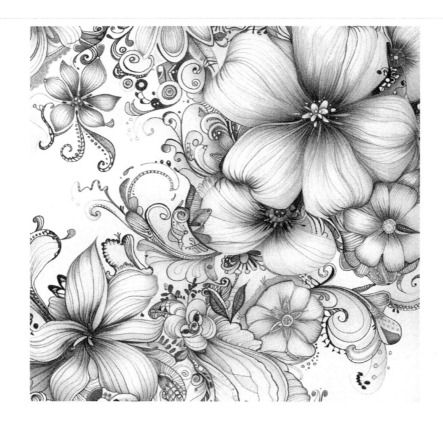

Sleep for Women's Health

Why This Impacts Sleep

- **Menstruation:** Due to changes in hormones, sleep may be impacted during menstruation. Disruptive side effects of periods, like cramps and mood swings, can influence your sleep during this time as well.

- **Pregnancy**: Pregnancy might cause discomfort, heartburn, and frequent urination, all things that may disrupt sleep.

- **Menopause**: Menopause can lead to hot flashes and insomnia, both common side effects of this time in a woman's life.

Specific Tips for Sleep

- Create a more comfortable environment during this period, and use things like heating pads or blankets to reduce any pain or discomfort.

- If you find you are hot or thirsty throughout the night, suck on ice chips. Keep a small cup in the freezer to prepare for this if needed. This is a better alternative to sipping water, which may keep you up frequently urinating throughout the night.

- Elevate your head during pregnancy if heartburn is causing discomfort at night. Exercise throughout the day to reduce menopause symptoms or period cramps.

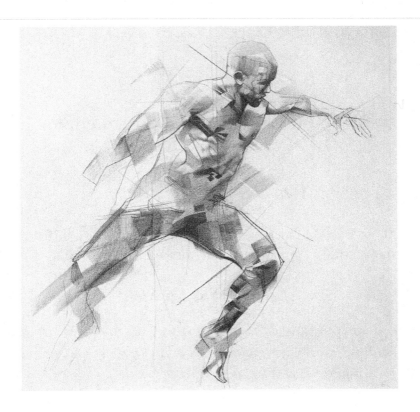

Sleep for Athletes

Why This Impacts Sleep

Athletes require more energy to sustain peak performance. Practices and games may make it difficult to find consistency in sleep schedules.

Specific Tips for Sleep

- Warm-up routines are important to incorporate into your routine as this will help improve performance and prepare you for the sporting events ahead. Incorporate them daily, even on days you won't be performing, to help regulate the body.

- After performing, ensure you allow time for your mind and muscles to relax. Take warm baths and do restful activities, such as reading or watching TV, while you recover.

- Eat foods rich in healthy carbohydrates for energy, and focus on lean proteins that will sustain energy during performance.

- Take naps to supplement energy on days of high performance.

Sleep for Non-Traditional Schedules

Why This Impacts Sleep

Those with unpredictable work schedules, who work second or third shifts, or who travel frequently might find that they struggle with jet lag and lethargy brought on by work.

Specific Tips for Sleep

- Invest in tools to help your body stay aligned with what an otherwise normal circadian rhythm would be. For example, use blackout curtains and eye masks to help induce darkness even if you have to sleep during the day.

- Create a consistent schedule with partners and roommates who might be helping with chores and caring for children. Even when schedules are unpredictable, doing things within the same range and window of time can be beneficial for maintaining a routine.

- When it comes to jet lag, try to follow a slow and gradual change leading up to the trip. Though you might not be able to do a total overhaul of your routine, small changes can prepare you to make the effects of jet lag less intense. Exercise on the first morning in the new time zone to help regulate your body and feel refreshed after travel.

- Use supplements during times of change to help your body adjust, in addition to other tools mentioned in Chapter 5.

Sleep for Those Over 60

Why This Impacts Sleep

Those who are over 60 might find that they suffer from more disruptions in their routine, leading to sleep disturbances. Due to less activity in older ages because of retirement or fewer responsibilities (like caring for children), those over 60 might find they have more energy late into the night.

Specific Tips for Sleep

- Avoid napping throughout the day. Instead, fill your day with mind-stimulating and energy-using activities that promote restfulness later on.

- Aim for at least seven hours of sleep per night and up to nine ("A Good Night's Sleep," n.d.)

- A helpful technique for those trying to fall asleep at night is to count up from 1 to 100. Imagine clouds and other soft images to help increase relaxation and focus.

After the implementation of the resources from this book, if you find your sleep is still troublesome, it may be a sign that you should consider seeking medical attention.

Conclusion

Sleep is so important to regulate, but many factors can contribute to poor sleep. By facilitating an environment in which you promote healthy sleep, you create the underpinnings for whole mind and body healing. In taking steps to improve your rest, you are taking steps to live a more peaceful life.

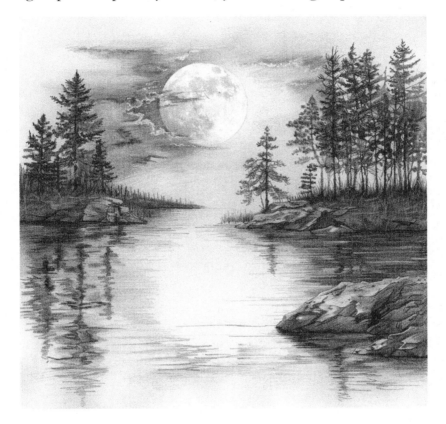

Sleep impacts *everything*. From the way you feel to how your body digests, your sleep habits might be the very thing that's making it so difficult for you to fall asleep at night. One night won't make or break your sleep health, but starting as soon as tonight, you could see improvements in your sleep. In the future, the thing that will make the most impact is your level of dedication and consistency to help facilitate an environment that promotes more restful nights.

If there's one thing to take away from this book, it's to not get overly anxious about bad sleep—this will ultimately create a cycle of stress that might be hard to escape from. Sleep health is important, and you will get to a place where you feel comfortable, confident, and more rested each night. You will likely have nights in the future where you wake up and can't fall back asleep, or maybe you can't even fall asleep in the first place. That's okay! Panicking will only make a small problem a big issue. This mindset alone can be enough to help get you started in the right direction with sleep health improvements.

Improving your sleep takes time and patience. Don't get discouraged if changes aren't immediate. Even once your sleep is regulated, it might still take time to see more positive results if you're making changes for things like digestion or hormonal balance. The body is strong and complex, meaning it's unlikely that you'll feel the full benefits right away. If after a few weeks, you are still struggling to get quality sleep, don't be afraid to reach out to a medical professional who can help rule out any other underlying health conditions that may be contributing to your poor sleep.

You will see improvements within a few weeks by following just a handful of the tips we've discussed in the previous chapters. Create a routine that works for you, and remember that everyone's bodies and needs are different. Even if you just get 10 more minutes of restful sleep a night, eventually, that will build into a solid nightly routine.

Check out the additional resources next to help further your exploration of sleep health. This is an ongoing health process, but it is very much worth the dedication!

Your Action Plan Recap

As a quick recap, remember the following steps for creating your perfect action plan going forward:

1. Understand sleep and why it's important to help boost motivation for positive change.

2. Establish the perfect routine to work with your body, and make adjustments along the way to help you find what's right.

3. Troubleshoot the challenges that disrupt your routine, and create boundaries with others to facilitate better sleep.

4. Create the ideal environment to get even more sleep and focus on elements like temperature and comfort to make your body happier each night.

5. Boost your sleep by adding additional elements for a more restful night in small increments to build a solid routine that lasts.

To help you take action and implement what you've learned in this book, use the 30-day Action Plan on the next page!

A Note From the Author

One of the best ways to learn about sleep health is by hearing about other people's experiences. Valuable sleep research comes from studying the patterns of people just like you!

To help keep the conversation around sleep going, please leave a review and share what you've struggled with and how you plan to overcome these setbacks. What did you learn that you will start to implement next? What has resonated the most?

Reviews are so important to helping make good books discoverable! Leaving one means a lot to my mission—to empower people with good-quality, actionable knowledge that improves health and well-being—and I'll be reading each one! Thank you for taking the time to submit a review, however short or long.

When sleep health is prioritized and managed, it can make a world of difference. This is good for your life, but also for your family, friends, and community! Spread the knowledge you've gained and leave a review to help spread the reach of this powerful insight.

***

If you enjoyed this book, you may enjoy other books by Dr Sui Wong – follow her on Amazon Author Central to receive alerts on new upcoming books!
https://www.amazon.com/author/drsuiwong

***

Continue your journey of improving your brain health & well-being with your next read from Dr Sui Wong's **Brain Health & Well-being Series:**

Mindfulness for Brain Health:

>> https://books2read.com/mindfulnessbrainhealth

In this book, I share practices for self-care to create Mindful Moments throughout the day. The book includes FREE audioguide meditations including practices to support better sleep.

Sweet Spot for Brain Health

>> **https://books2read.com/sweet-spot-brain-health**

Sweet Spot for Brain Health is your ultimate guide to manage your sugar levels for improved mental clarity, focus, productivity and well-being.

Inside, you'll find

- **extensively researched, science-backed information on the brain-glucose connection, with insights into the basics of brain metabolism and how different energy sources impact cognitive function.**
- powerful tools for blood glucose management
- **how intermittent fasting can improve metabolic flexibility and practical tips to do this**
- practical nutrition strategies that you can implement immediately.
- tips to satisfy your sweet tooth while staying healthy, so you need not go completely sugar-free!
- **expert advice on lifestyle practices that balance blood sugar and enhance your brain health**
- **a bonus 12-week challenge**, where you can apply the valuable knowledge you've gained for a sustainable, healthy lifestyle.

And much more.

30 Days to Better Sleep

You deserve a quality night's sleep every single day! Using this 30-day plan, you'll empower yourself to do just that. Over the next 30 days, there are three essential things you can do to improve sleep quality:

1. Establish a solid morning routine to create consistency.

2. Establish a solid nightly routine to reinforce that consistency.

3. Improve your overall quality of sleep so each night you feel more rested.

The next 30 days will be broken down into these 3 phases, with a daily goal to help you achieve consistency in your routine. Each day, you'll repeat the goals from the previous days, helping you find a more restful sleep at the end of the 30 days.

In the lefthand column, you'll find a daily goal. Then, on the right, there is space for you to reflect on this goal. Consider the challenges, benefits, motivations, or intentions of the goal and reflect on this in your own words in the space provided.

Sleep Tracker

Before diving into the next 30 days of better sleep, you'll find a table below to help track your sleep routine, enabling you to be more aware of your sleep habits so you can make changes as needed.

Instructions:

1. Write the day of the week (Monday-Sunday) in the first column, followed by the date in the second.

2. Next, write down when you went to bed (ie. 10:30 p.m., 12:00 a.m., etc.) and when you woke up in the column after that. Pick a time that works for your schedule and try to stick to this every day.

3. Write down any minutes spent napping that day. Aim to limit your nap to 30 minutes and try napping only in the early afternoon to prevent naps from affecting nighttime sleepiness.

4. In the quality column, rate how you felt this quality of sleep was on a scale of 1-10.

5. Lastly, write an overall feeling rating from 1-10, considering how your mind and body felt throughout the day.

This will help you notice any influences in your quality of sleep as well as provide a point for you to see the positive growth or change you've experienced.

Note: After keeping to a regular schedule for two weeks, if you still feel consistently tired, increase the amount of sleep slightly, like by going to bed 30 minutes earlier. Keep to that new regular schedule to help determine the optimal duration of sleep needed.

Day:	Date:	Bedtime:	When Woke Up:	I Total Time	Nap	Quality Rating	Feeling Rating

Phase 1: Find Your Morning Routine

Day 1 Goal	Reflection
Reflect on your sleep patterns, and what main goals you have to improve sleep quality.	
Day 2 Goal	**Reflection**
Choose a specific time to wake up each day. Ensure you give yourself enough time to get ready in the morning. Begin waking up at the same time each day going forward—even the weekend.	
Day 3 Goal	**Reflection**
Counting back from this wake time, set a specific bedtime to follow each day. Refer to Chapter 2 if you need help creating a routine.	
Day 4 Goal	**Reflection**
Focus on your ideal bed and wake time, and identify the main obstacles that can make it challenging to follow this routine.	
Day 5 Goal	**Reflection**
Create a list of reminders as to why this consistent bed and wake time is important to you, and use it as motivation to stay on top of your routine. Refer to Chapter 1 to learn more about the importance of healthy sleep.	
Day 6 Goal	**Reflection**
Incorporate bright light in your morning routine to see how this can help wake you up and provide a sense of alertness. See Chapter 2 to learn more about how light impacts sleep.	

Day 7 Goal	Reflection
Reflect on your progress so far. What changes can you implement to stay consistent with this routine?	

Day 8 Goal	Reflection
Set a fitness goal to get a certain amount of exercise each morning, starting with 10 minutes a day and adjusting as needed to fit your schedule. Refer to Chapter 2's Physical Activity Guide as needed.	

Day 9 Goal	Reflection
Keep following your ideal routine, and supplement with naps as needed. **Remember**: keep naps to 30 minutes and only take them in the early afternoon.	

Day 10 Goal	Reflection
Look at your morning routine and identify how well you've been following this routine. Make any needed adjustments, and continue following this new routine.	

Phase 2: Establish a Nightly Routine

Day 11 Goal	Reflection
Identify your perfect bedtime. Make needed adjustments to this bedtime, and do your best to continue to follow your consistent routine.	

Day 12 Goal	Reflection
Incorporate a nightly relaxation breathing exercise into your routine (see Chapter 2 for more information on breathing exercises).	

Day 13 Goal	Reflection
Set a goal to limit caffeine at least 12 hours before bed.	

Day 14 Goal	Reflection
Add a light stretch routine to your nightly breathing exercises.	

Day 15 Goal	Reflection
Since you are halfway through the 30 days to better sleep, reflect on your sleep tracker and notice any patterns or habits that may be disrupting your sleep.	

Day 16 Goal	Reflection
Continue to follow the same routine and experiment with different stretches and breathing exercises (see chapter 2 for more information).	

Day 17 Goal	Reflection
Create a new self-care goal to incorporate something into your nightly routine, such as reading or a skincare regimen.	

Day 18 Goal	Reflection
Practice meditation for at least 10 minutes before bed tonight.	

Day 19 Goal	Reflection
Identify the main successes you've had with establishing a morning and nightly routine, and how this has made you feel.	

Day 20 Goal	Reflection
Reflect on your routine as well as the sleep tracker and write down some of your strengths and weaknesses you notice.	

Phase 3: Improve Sleep Quality

Day 21 Goal	Reflection
Reflect on your changes in sleep quality based on setting an established routine.	

Day 22 Goal	Reflection
Create a new goal to improve quality even further. Write down the steps you will need to take to reach this goal, and what will motivate you to get there.	

Day 23 Goal	Reflection
Incorporate something in your daily routine that will improve sleep quality, such as mindfulness, stretching, or journaling.	

Day 24 Goal	Reflection
Celebrate your successes so far, and thank yourself for putting in work to get better sleep.	

Day 25 Goal	Reflection
Identify the biggest challenges you will face going forward, and what you can do to overcome those challenges.	

Day 26 Goal	Reflection
Continue to follow the same routine, and reflect on what you've learned through this experience.	

Day 27 Goal	Reflection
Look back on your sleep tracker and identify one thing that negatively impacted your sleep routine the most. Refer to Chapters 3 and 4 to see if any of these disturbances have been keeping you awake.	

Day 28 Goal	Reflection
Keep practicing the same routine, and highlight the positive changes you've experienced.	

Day 29 Goal	Reflection
Identify what has positively changed the most about how you feel physically and mentally after these 30 days.	

Day 30 Goal	Reflection
Celebrate making it to the last day, and continue to follow your routine going forward. Share this plan with someone else, and consider repeating the above with someone to make continuous progress and to help encourage others to get better sleep!	

Transform Lives Through Better Sleep

Your Experience Can Change Someone's Life

"The first wealth is health." - Ralph Waldo Emerson

Now that you have everything you need to transform your sleep and boost your daily energy, you can help others find their path to better rest too.

Did you know that many people struggle to find reliable information about sleep? They face the same challenges you might have experienced - feeling tired all the time, having trouble falling asleep, or waking up feeling groggy. Your honest review could help them discover the solutions they're looking for.

As a neurologist, my mission is to help everyone understand how to get the rest they need to live their best life. But to reach more people who need this information, I need your help.

Your review could help: ...one more tired parent get the rest they need to care for their family ...one more student succeed in school by sleeping better ...one more worker feel energized and focused at their job ...one more person break free from their sleep struggles ...one more life transform through better sleep habits

The science of sleep becomes more powerful when we share what works. Your experience could be exactly what someone else needs to hear to start their journey toward better sleep.

To make a difference, simply follow this link or scan the QR code to leave a review on your local Amazon marketplace:

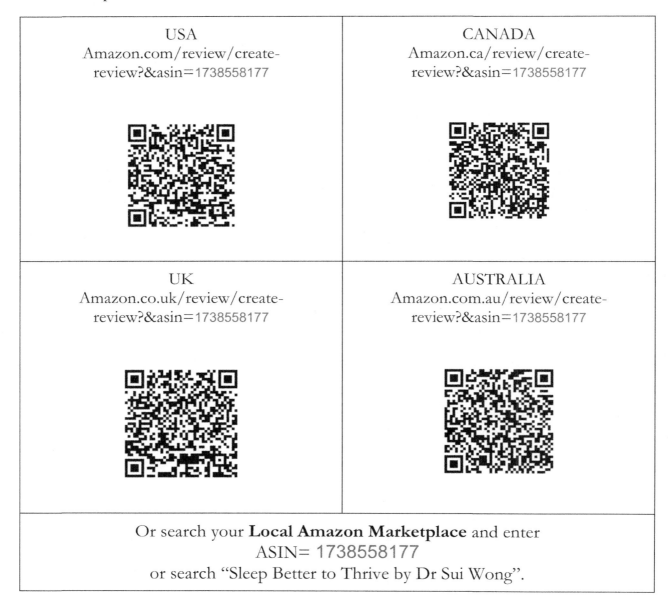

USA	CANADA
Amazon.com/review/create-review?&asin=1738558177	Amazon.ca/review/create-review?&asin=1738558177

UK	AUSTRALIA
Amazon.co.uk/review/create-review?&asin=1738558177	Amazon.com.au/review/create-review?&asin=1738558177

Or search your **Local Amazon Marketplace** and enter
ASIN= 1738558177
or search "Sleep Better to Thrive by Dr Sui Wong".

Thank you for helping others find their path to better sleep. Your kindness in sharing your thoughts means the world to me and to all the future readers you'll help.

With gratitude, Dr. Sui Wong

P.S. Just like quality sleep makes everything better, your review could make someone's journey to better sleep easier!

Additional Sleep Resources

Below are some resources that may help you continue the process of building a better sleep routine.

Specialized Help

At times, you may find that you would benefit from more specialized help. There are a few conditions that you might find are preventing you from getting a good night's sleep. These include:

- sleep apnea

- narcolepsy

- restless leg syndrome

- night terrors

To help you determine if you might be struggling with any of these conditions, talk to a medical professional. You can also find help from accredited websites like The Cleveland Clinic or Johns Hopkins Medicine.

Continued Learning

Below are a few suggested books and podcast to help you continue your journey of sleep improvement:

- ***The 4 Pillar Plan*** *by Dr. Rangan Chatterjee*

- **Why We Sleep: Unlocking the Power of Sleep and Dreams** *by Matthew Walker*

- **Huberman Lab Podcast** *Guest Series | Dr. Matt Walker*

Online Sources

- Center for Human Sleep Science

  - www.humansleepscience.com

- Sleep Foundation

  - www.sleepfoundation.org

- National Sleep Foundation

  - www.thensf.org

Lastly, check out my website drsuiwongmd.com, where you can sign up for my mailing list, and sign up on bit.ly/sleepbetterbonuses to download free worksheets, and find a Yoga Nidra (yogic sleep) audio! On top of this, you'll discover more tools to help support more cognitive abilities to leave a positive impact on your mind and body.

Appendix

For downloadable templates and worksheets from this book, sign up at bit.ly/sleepbetterbonuses

Follow me on Amazon Author Central to receive alerts on new upcoming books!
https://www.amazon.com/author/drsuiwong

Thursday Tips! Get my popular Thursday Tips [TT] where I share bite- size brain health tips to thrive – a 1-min read with 3 tips and 1 question! – sign up via **bit.ly/drwongbrainhealth**

Get alerts on upcoming book releases, via **bit.ly/drwongbrainhealth**

Other books you may enjoy:

These books are available on Amazon as paperback, e-book, and audiobook:
Mindfulness for Brain Health: **https://books2read.com/mindfulnessbrainhealth**

Sweet Spot for Brain Health:

https://books2read.com/sweet-spot-brain-health

Quit Ultra-Processed Foods Now: **https://books2read.com/quitupf**

References

The references provided here include a mixture of scientific articles and websites that provide valuable information and that you can easily access to do further reading. Keep in mind that new studies are constantly being conducted. You can use the resources here to help you build your knowledge base and take your health journey into your own hands.

A good night's sleep. (n.d.). NIH. https://www.nia.nih.gov/health/sleep/good-nights-sleep

Abbasi-Feinberg, F., Aurora, R. N., Carden, K. A., Kapur, V. K., Malhotra, R. K., Martin, J. L., Olson, E. J., Ramar, K., Rosen, C. L., Rowley, J. A., Shelgikar, A. V., Trotti, L. M. (2021, October 1). *Sleep is essential to health: an American Academy of Sleep Medicine position statement.* JCSM. https://jcsm.aasm.org/doi/full/10.5664/jcsm.9476

Alshobaili, F. & AlYousefi, N. (2019, June 8). *The effect of smartphone usage at bedtime on sleep quality among Saudi non-medical staff at King Saud University Medical City.* National Library of Medicine. https://www.ncbi.nlm.nih.gov/pmc/articles/PMC6618184/

Baron, E. D., Cooper, K. D., Koo, B., Matsui, M. S., Oyetakin-White, P., Suggs, A., Yarosh, D. (2014, September 30). *Does poor sleep quality affect skin aging?* National Library of Medicine. https://pubmed.ncbi.nlm.nih.gov/25266053/

Benton, D., Bloxham, A., Brennan, A., Gaylor, C., Young, H. A. (2022, September 21). *Carbohydrate and sleep: an evaluation of putative mechanisms.* NIH. https://www.ncbi.nlm.nih.gov/pmc/articles/PMC9532617/

Blume, C., Garbazza, C., & Spitschan, M. (2019, August 20). *Effects of light on human circadian rhythms, sleep, and mood.* NIH. https://www.ncbi.nlm.nih.gov/pmc/articles/PMC6751071/

Bryan, L. (2023, December 14). *Adenosine and sleep: understanding your sleep drive.* The Sleep Foundation. https://www.sleepfoundation.org/how-sleep-works/adenosine-and-sleep

Bryan, L. (2024a, April 5). *Why do we need sleep?* The Sleep Foundation. https://www.sleepfoundation.org/how-sleep-works/why-do-we-need-sleep

Bryan, L. (2024b, March 15). *Circadian rhythm.* The Sleep Foundation. https://www.sleepfoundation.org/circadian-rhythm

Bryan, L. (2024c, May 7). *Alcohol and sleep.* The Sleep Foundation. https://www.sleepfoundation.org/nutrition/alcohol-and-sleep

Carollo, M. (2024, April 10). *Reduce stress through decluttering*. Columbia University Irving Medical Center. https://www.columbiadoctors.org/news/reduce-stress-through-decluttering

Cat keeping you awake? How to manage night activity. (n.d.). Animal Humane Society. https://www.animalhumanesociety.org/resource/cat-keeping-you-awake-how-manage-night-activity

Chesak, J. (2023, March 20). *How these 3 sleep positions affect your gut health*. Healthline. https://www.healthline.com/health/healthy-sleep/sleep-effects-digestion

Dasgupta, R. (2021, September 1). *How sleep can affect your hormone levels, plus 12 ways to sleep deep*. Healthline. https://www.healthline.com/health/sleep/how-sleep-can-affect-your-hormone-levels

Davis, N. (2019, December 11). *The best workout routine to do before bedtime*. Healthline. https://www.healthline.com/health/sleep/the-best-workout-routine-to-do-before-bedtime

Dinardo, K. (2020, October 10). *Rest better with light exercises*. The New York Times. https://www.nytimes.com/2020/10/10/at-home/exercises-for-better-sleep.html

Everett, A. C., Hinko, A., Horowitz, J. F., Newsom, S. A. (2013, August 13). *A single session of low-intensity exercise Is sufficient to enhance insulin sensitivity into the next day in obese adults*. National Library of Medicine. https://www.ncbi.nlm.nih.gov/pmc/articles/PMC3747878/

Foods that help you sleep. (2020, December). The Sleep Charity. https://thesleepcharity.org.uk/information-support/adults/sleep-hub/foods-that-help-you-sleep/

Good sleep for good health. (2021, April). News in Health. https://newsinhealth.nih.gov/2021/04/good-sleep-good-health

Gupta, S., Shankar, E., & Srivastava, J. (2011, February 1). *Chamomile: A herbal medicine of the past with bright future*. NIH. https://www.ncbi.nlm.nih.gov/pmc/articles/PMC2995283/

Hong, S., Jeong, J., & Kim, T. (2015, March 11). *The impact of sleep and circadian disturbance on hormones and metabolism*. National Library of Medicine. https://www.ncbi.nlm.nih.gov/pmc/articles/PMC4377487/

Hormones. (2022, February 23). The Cleveland Clinic. https://my.clevelandclinic.org/health/articles/22464-hormones

How sleep deprivation impacts mental health. (2022, March 16). Columbia University Irving Medical Center. https://www.columbiapsychiatry.org/news/how-sleep-deprivation-affects-your-mental-health

Human growth hormone (HGH). (2022, June 21). The Cleveland Clinic. https://my.clevelandclinic.org/health/articles/23309-human-growth-hormone-hgh

Insomnia. (n.d.). The Cleveland Clinic. https://my.clevelandclinic.org/health/diseases/12119-insomnia

Koala fact sheet. (2020, July 1). PBS. https://www.pbs.org/wnet/nature/blog/koala-fact-sheet/

Krans, B. (2018, August 17). *Foods that can improve sleep.* Healthline. https://www.healthline.com/health/foods-for-better-sleep

Martin, W. (2023, March 15). *Why morning people should never teach or grade after 6 p.m.* Harvard Business Publishing. https://hbsp.harvard.edu/inspiring-minds/why-morning-people-should-never-teach-or-grade-after-6-p-m

McTigue, S. (2020, February 27). *Do babies sleep in the womb?* Healthline. https://www.healthline.com/health/pregnancy/do-babies-sleep-in-the-womb

Newsom, R. (2023, November 1). *Nicotine and sleep.* The Sleep Foundation. https://www.sleepfoundation.org/physical-health/nicotine-and-sleep

Newsom, R. (2024a, January 12). *Blue light: what it is and how it affects sleep.* The Sleep Foundation. https://www.sleepfoundation.org/bedroom-environment/blue-light

Newsom, R. (2024b, May 7). *Cognitive behavioral therapy for insomnia (CBT-I): An overview.* The Sleep Foundation. https://www.sleepfoundation.org/insomnia/treatment/cognitive-behavioral-therapy-insomnia

Pacheco, D. (2023, October 26). *Sleep and blood glucose levels.* The Sleep Foundation. https://www.sleepfoundation.org/physical-health/sleep-and-blood-glucose-levels

Pacheco, D. (2024a, April 11). *Sleep inertia: how to combat morning grogginess.* The Sleep Foundation. https://www.sleepfoundation.org/how-sleep-works/sleep-inertia

Pacheco, D. (2024b, April 17). *Caffeine and sleep.* The Sleep Foundation. https://www.sleepfoundation.org/nutrition/caffeine-and-sleep

Pacheco, D. (2024c, March 7). *Best temperature for sleep.* The Sleep Foundation. https://www.sleepfoundation.org/bedroom-environment/best-temperature-for-sleep

Pacheco, D. (2024d, May 13). *How to become a morning person.* The Sleep Foundation. https://www.sleepfoundation.org/sleep-faqs/how-to-become-a-morning-person

Peters, B. (2023, May 22). *Is eating before bed bad for you?* Verywell Health. https://www.verywellhealth.com/eating-before-bed-3014981

Rausch-Phung, E., & Rehman, A. (2023, December 19). *How long should it take to fall asleep?* The Sleep Foundation. https://www.sleepfoundation.org/sleep-faqs/how-long-should-it-take-to-fall-asleep

Rosen, L. (2015, August 31). *Relax, turn off your phone, and go to sleep*. Harvard Business Review. https://hbr.org/2015/08/research-shows-how-anxiety-and-technology-are-affecting-our-sleep

Salamon, M. (2022, November 16). *How blue light affects your sleep*. WebMD. https://www.webmd.com/sleep-disorders/sleep-blue-light

Sheikh, Z. (2023, November 13). *Foods high in tryptophan*. WebMD. https://www.webmd.com/diet/foods-high-in-tryptophan

Sleep. (2023, June 19). The Cleveland Clinic. https://my.clevelandclinic.org/health/body/12148-sleep-basics

Sleep. (n.d.). American Heart Association. https://www.heart.org/en/healthy-living/healthy-lifestyle/sleep

Sleep Needs, Patterns, and Difficulties of Adolescents: Summary of a Workshop. (2000). NIH. https://www.ncbi.nlm.nih.gov/books/NBK222804/

Stanborough, R. J. (2020, July 10). *How does cortisol affect your sleep?* Healthline. https://www.healthline.com/health/cortisol-and-sleep

Stress and sleep. (n.d.). American Psychological Association. https://www.apa.org/news/press/releases/stress/2013/sleep

Summer, J. (2024a, April 19). *What is tryptophan?* The Sleep Foundation. https://www.sleepfoundation.org/nutrition/what-is-tryptophan

Summer, J. (2024b, February 29). *8 health benefits of sleep*. The Sleep Foundation. https://www.sleepfoundation.org/how-sleep-works/benefits-of-sleep

Summer, J. (2024c, March 11). *Napping: benefits and tips*. The Sleep Foundation. https://www.sleepfoundation.org/napping

Summer, J. (2024d, March 7). *How noise can affect your sleep satisfaction*. The Sleep Foundation. https://www.sleepfoundation.org/noise-and-sleep

Suni, E. (2023a, December 21). *How do animals sleep?* The Sleep Foundation. https://www.sleepfoundation.org/animals-and-sleep

Suni, E. (2023b, July 18). *How lack of sleep impacts cognitive performance and focus*. The Sleep Foundation. https://www.sleepfoundation.org/sleep-deprivation/lack-of-sleep-and-cognitive-impairment

Suni, E. (2023c, June 1). *Myths and facts about sleep*. The Sleep Foundation. https://www.sleepfoundation.org/how-sleep-works/myths-and-facts-about-sleep

Suni, E. (2024a, April 10). *Best sleeping positions.* The Sleep Foundation. https://www.sleepfoundation.org/sleeping-positions

Suni, E. (2024b, April 12). *The best foods to help you sleep.* The Sleep Foundation. https://www.sleepfoundation.org/nutrition/food-and-drink-promote-good-nights-sleep

Suni, E. (2024c, March 27). *Insomnia: symptoms, causes, and treatments.* The Sleep Foundation. https://www.sleepfoundation.org/insomnia

Suni, E. (2024d, May 13). *How much sleep do you need?* The Sleep Foundation. https://www.sleepfoundation.org/how-sleep-works/how-much-sleep-do-we-really-need

The best times to eat. (2023, October). Northwestern Medicine. https://www.nm.org/healthbeat/healthy-tips/nutrition/best-times-to-eat

The state of sleep health in America 2023. (n.d.). American Sleep Apnea Association. https://www.sleephealth.org/sleep-health/the-state-of-sleephealth-in-america/

Vandekerckhove, M. (2017, December 1). *Emotion, emotion regulation, and sleep: an intimate relationship.* NIH. https://www.ncbi.nlm.nih.gov/pmc/articles/PMC7181893/

Walker, M. (n.d.). *The buzz on alcohol and caffeine.* Master Class. https://www.masterclass.com/classes/matthew-walker-teaches-the-science-of-better-sleep/chapters/the-buzz-on-alcohol-and-caffeine

Watson, K. (2023, February 10). *How long does it take for water to pass through your body?* Healthline. https://www.healthline.com/health/digestive-health/how-long-does-it-take-for-water-to-pass-through-your-body

What to wear to bed: pajamas, socks or nothing at all. (2023, April 25). The Better Sleep Council. https://bettersleep.org/blog/what-to-wear-to-bed-pajamas-socks-or-nothing-at-all/

Why is sleep important. (n.d.). American Psychological Association. https://www.apa.org/topics/sleep/why

Why is sleep important? (2022, March 24). NIH. https://www.nhlbi.nih.gov/health/sleep/why-sleep-important

Why sleep matters: benefits of sleep. (2021, October 1). Division of Sleep Medicine. https://sleep.hms.harvard.edu/education-training/public-education/sleep-and-health-education-program/sleep-health-education-41

Image Reference:

I created the illustrations in this book using Midjourney www.midjourney.com. I am grateful for this tool that helped me bring forth my vision for these images.

Printed in Great Britain
by Amazon

56403410R00057